THE ICE BUCKET CHALLENGE

CASEY SHERMAN & DAVE WEDGE

THE ICE BUCKET CHALLENGE

PETE FRATES AND THE
FIGHT AGAINST ALS

ForeEdge

ForeEdge
An imprint of University Press of New England
www.upne.com
© 2017 Casey Sherman and Dave Wedge
All rights reserved
Manufactured in the United States of America
Designed by Mindy Basinger Hill
Typeset in Minion Pro

For permission to reproduce any of the material in this book,
contact Permissions, University Press of New England, One Court Street,
Suite 250, Lebanon NH 03766; or visit www.upne.com

Library of Congress Cataloging-in-Publication Data available upon request

Paperback ISBN: 978-1-5126-0096-4
Ebook ISBN: 978-1-5126-0159-6

5   4   3   2   1

FOR BELLA AND MIA: the best daughters
a dad could ever ask for.
Stay compassionate and dedicated
Casey Sherman

FOR DANIELLE AND JACKSON: ever to excel
Dave Wedge

CONTENTS

Illustrations follow page 96

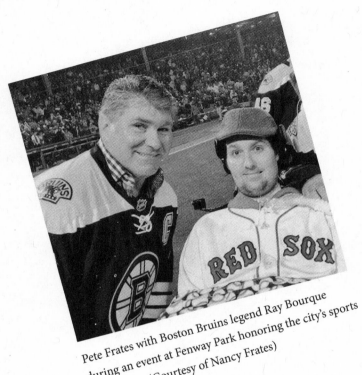

Pete Frates with Boston Bruins legend Ray Bourque during an event at Fenway Park honoring the city's sports champions. (Courtesy of Nancy Frates)

FOREWORD

I first met Pete Frates in 2012, when he refereed a charity "old timers" game I was playing in with several fellow Boston Bruins alumni. It was just a brief encounter, and it didn't really stand out at the time, but soon I would come to know just who Pete was and exactly what he represented.

A few months after that chance meeting at the hockey rink, Pete was told something that no one should ever hear, especially a healthy twenty-seven-year-old athlete with his whole life ahead of him. He was told by his doctors that he had ALS, also known as Lou Gehrig's disease, and that his condition was terminal.

While the diagnosis was certainly a devastating blow, for Pete it wasn't the end.

It was only the beginning.

Before Pete Frates, ALS was just another mysterious disease that people knew only if they had a family member afflicted by it or if they had read about Lou Gehrig's heart-wrenching story. While many other diseases had well-funded awareness campaigns and global organizations to raise millions of dollars for scientific research, dedicated ALS warriors were in need of a fearless leader.

In stepped Pete and the world soon took notice.

It didn't take long before we all became motivated and inspired by this young man's strength, courage, perseverance, and drive not only to fight a disease but to alter the course of history through the immense power and global reach of social media. Pete took the tenacity, passion, intensity, and dedication that he exhibited in the rinks and on the ball fields as a star athlete and channeled his energy into fighting the disease that was invading his body.

I've had the privilege of getting to know Pete and his amazing family over the past few years and have shared many incredible moments with them, whether attending an ALS fund-raiser or a sports ceremony or simply relaxing while watching our beloved Boston Bruins battle at the Boston Garden. Every moment with them and with Pete has been a blessing.

This book, written by acclaimed authors and journalists Casey Sherman and Dave Wedge, is not one of sadness or tragedy. Instead, it's one of love and hope. It's the story not only of a man who decided to live his life to the fullest while staring down a death sentence but also of a man who took that grim reality and used it to create an instantly memorable, creative, and impactful way to raise ALS awareness.

I'm not even sure if Pete knew how big the Ice Bucket Challenge would get, but one thing is for sure: because of Pete, the world knows a lot more about the ALS fight today than ever before, and a cure for this horrific disease is finally within reach. Pete's viral campaign showed the true power of social media and proved that something as simple as an iPhone and a bucket of icy water could change the world.

Pete loves his Boston sports teams, and as a kid he looked up to a lot of pro athletes, including me. But to me and to so many others, he's the real role model. To witness his courage and resilience, and his family's grace, has been one of the great gifts of my life. I will forever be grateful to have had the great fortune of getting to know such a brave and inspiring figure.

RAY BOURQUE *former Boston Bruins captain and member of the NHL Hall of Fame*

PROLOGUE

CAPE CORAL, FLORIDA
AUGUST 23, 2011

Pete Frates popped the top of an ice-cold Corona and handed it to his mother, Nancy, before reaching for one of his own. They lifted their beer bottles in salute of what had been the perfect Florida getaway vacation. The scorching sun of mid-afternoon had finally burned off, and now there was a light breeze coming off the ocean. Nancy's husband, John, was inside the house fixing a ceiling fan with their oldest daughter, Jenn. Pete and his mother left them to it. Instead they chose to take a late afternoon swim in the backyard pool. They were on vacation, after all.

Lounging on a float, Pete glistened in the water, his chiseled features, bright white smile, and dark summer tan standing out against the colorful sky. Another summer of city league baseball, coupled with his usual intense workout regimen, had him in tip-top shape. He was enjoying this last vacation moment, as the next day he and the family were heading back to Boston for a playoff game for Pete's team, the Lexington Blue Sox. The family would also be meeting Pete's new girlfriend, Julie, a Boston College senior whom Pete had been dating for a few months.

Pete had always been an outgoing guy with a sharp wit and a thirst for fun. He had strong opinions about a host of topics, including sports, music, and politics, and was not shy about sharing them with his buddies. But he could also be reflective at times. He shared a special bond with his parents and felt he could talk to them about virtually anything that was on his mind. With eyes closed under a pair of dark shades, he continued to float, seemingly lost in thought. Suddenly, he spoke. "I'm thinking about leaving my job," he announced abruptly, breaking the serenity of the moment and surprising his mother.

Pete had been working for Humana as a health-insurance broker for the past two years, and Nancy knew it was not what he wanted to do. But still, it was a steady job in a down economy. She gave him a concerned look. He shrugged and took a pull from his beer. "I'm not passionate about it," he explained. "I'm supposed to be doing something else."

Nancy analyzed his words as only a mother can do. He has a new girlfriend, an apartment in South Boston, a car payment, and other bills. How was he going to make a living? "How are you going to do this Pete?" she asked.

He did not have a plan. What he did have was a hunch. "It's not anything I'm going to jump into," he replied. "But I just think I'm meant for something else. I'm not sure this is what I'm supposed to be doing."

Nancy took a practical approach to her son's dilemma. "You can't quit your job unless you have another one," she said.

Pete took off his sunglasses and gave his mother a serious look. She did not understand what he was trying to tell her. He was not interested in another job. What he wanted was a mission.

Nancy stared into her son's eyes and recognized that he was at a personal crossroads. "But, Pete," she offered softly, "you have to follow your passion. You have to be happy. You can't begrudge every morning you wake up and not be passionate about what you're doing."

"I know, Mom," he said. "I know." His voice trailed off and he floated in the silence for a moment. He looked up at the sky, the sun illuminating his wet face. He paused, turned toward his mother, and gave her a smile. He climbed out of the pool, put down his beer, and dove back into the water, swimming the length of the pool.

It was all but settled at that moment. Pete Frates's life was about to change. He just did not know how.

THE ICE BUCKET CHALLENGE

1

THE BATTER'S BOX

Julie Kowalik sat quietly at the kitchen island of her childhood home in the quaint, coastal town of Marblehead, Massachusetts, while her mother tried vainly to engage her in conversation. Julie nodded as her mom spoke, but she was not paying attention to the words, as she was having her own dialogue in her mind. Kate Kowalik recognized immediately that her daughter's thoughts had drifted to the new man in her life.

"Well, how serious is this?" Kate asked.

"I'm a little nervous," Julie admitted sheepishly. She had been dating Pete Frates for only a few months, but tonight she and a friend were set to get on a bus in South Boston with a group of Pete's closest friends. It would be the first night that she would truly enter Pete's world. Julie, now heading into her senior year as an economics major at Boston College, had gone shopping earlier in the day and bought a new skirt and top that would show off her golden summer tan. She went to her bedroom and looked at herself again in the mirror.

How do you dress for a baseball game when we're going out after? Julie asked herself. *Am I overdressed for a baseball game?* She was faced with a fashion challenge. Julie wanted to look attractive for her boyfriend, but she also understood that Pete's parents, John and Nancy, would be there. She examined her new outfit in the mirror once again. *Definitely nothing too tight or risqué,* she thought.

Julie had only met them briefly before, but she and Pete were getting serious, and she was determined to make a good impression. She settled on a white, strapless summer dress that revealed her browned shoulders and back, but she threw on a little jean jacket. She told herself it was in case she got cold, but really it was to lower the dress's *wow* factor for Pete's parents.

Nancy and John flew into Boston that morning after their relaxing vacation in Cape Coral. The night before they left, the family took a photo together on the water underneath the soft red hues of the Gulf Coast sunset. The Frates were blessed and they knew it. Nancy stared at the photo taken with her cell phone and saw the perfect family—two handsome sons, a beautiful daughter, and she and her husband. They were two proud parents who had been on a journey filled with peaks and valleys in an effort to provide a foundation of emotional, financial, and moral support for their kids.

They had returned home to watch Pete perform in the Boston City League play-offs. It was a competitive league made up of former college baseball stars that were no longer playing for a scholarship or a minor league contract but now took the field simply for the love of the game.

Nancy felt anxious as she and John left their house and drove twenty minutes to the ball field. She was about to spend some quality time with Pete's new girlfriend, and she too was nervous. Nancy hoped to make a good impression on the young woman because she had a warm feeling about Julie. Pete certainly had no shortage of girlfriends over the years, but none before had taken any real interest in baseball. To Nancy, sports were a true window into her son's soul.

"She must really like him," she said to John. "She's the first girl we'll meet at one of his baseball games."

"I wish he'd find someone and get married," John responded, only half-joking. "But he is married actually—to baseball."

Julie and her friend Elise DePrisco were also on the road, making the winding drive down the rugged Atlantic Ocean coastline from Marblehead to Boston. They parked outside Pete's apartment on D Street in South Boston, a neighborhood once home to notorious crime boss James "Whitey" Bulger. But the area had changed over time, transforming itself from a rough-and-tumble, predominantly Irish working-class district into a gentrified playground for young twenty-something professionals looking for fun, love, and city living.

Inside Pete's apartment, the beer flowed as his friends and their girl-friends sized up Julie and Elise. Pete's buddies were all trying to make their marks in the real world. They all had real responsibilities. Julie still lived in a college dorm. They wondered why Pete had fallen so hard for this young coed.

She was attractive for sure. A real head-turner. Julie had natural blond hair that flowed over her shoulders and bounced when she walked. She had bright, inquisitive eyes; an infectious smile; and an athletic body. But Pete's friends knew that good looks only went so far. This new girl must be different.

Julie felt all eyes on her and she did not have Pete there to lean on. He was already warming up at the ball field with his team. Julie was left virtually alone in the lion's den of Pete's social circle. She struggled a bit through forced, awkward conversation but tried not to let her nerves show. Julie fielded question after question, most posed by the other girlfriends. She felt like she was on a job interview—albeit one with Jell-O shots and beer-filled red Solo cups.

Julie and Elise joined Pete's friends as they boarded a party bus and were driven to Pine Banks Field in nearby Melrose. The group gathered on a grassy knoll near right field to cheer on Pete.

As Nancy and John Frates arrived at the field, they made their way to the outfield party to meet Julie. The floodlights illuminating the ball field shone brightly, reflecting off the green grass and the youthful, smiling faces of Pete's many friends. Someone handed Nancy and John cold beers. Friends sat on coolers, others on blankets. It reminded Nancy and John of the many football tailgates at their alma mater, Boston College, where they had fallen in love so many years before.

They saw Julie, her sun-streaked blond hair and dark tan contrasting with her wide, bright smile, as she laughed with Elise. She turned and saw them, smiled, and strode over. Julie and Nancy instinctively hugged. She smiled again and hugged John. There was an immediate comfort level and bond between Pete's parents and Julie. They felt like they had already known her for years.

"How's it going with this crew?" John asked, gesturing to a group of Pete's rowdy friends.

Julie laughed. "Nothing I can't handle. I'm a BC girl, remember."

"Well it's so good of you to come to one of Pete's games, especially with all these shenanigans," Nancy said.

"It's fun!" Julie said. "I like his friends."

She introduced them to Elise and they shared a beer under the lights as the game got underway. Nancy and John hugged her again and figured they would go watch the game and let the kids have their party. Normally, they always sat along one of the baselines to watch Pete play. They liked to do that because Pete would always stop and talk to them as he walked to and from the dugout. But this night, as they walked back from the outfield toward where they were planning to sit, Pete came up to bat, so they decided to grab the first seats they found and watch him hit. It happened to be right behind home plate—somewhere they rarely sat for his games.

As Pete got ready in the dugout, he heard his family and friends howling and cheering from the outfield. He knew Julie was there to see him play and would have been lying to himself if he did not admit he was equally nervous to impress her. Typically, there were only some parents and a few girlfriends at the games, although play-off games were a bit more crowded. Pete's robust personal cheering section had his adrenaline pumping hard.

The Lexington Blue Sox, Pete's team, was facing their rival, the Andre Chiefs. Most of the league's players knew one another and had played together or against one another in college. Now they were out of school and forced to grow up and get jobs, as their parents had done before them. Still, there was a competitive fire that burned in each player, players who refused to let go of their passionate youths.

Pete was at his physical peak. He was twenty-six-years-old and running thirteen miles a day at a six minute-per-mile clip. He was doing a hundred push-ups a minute and thirty pull-ups a minute and bench pressing three-hundred-plus pounds.

He had just performed beyond his own expectations at a Tough Mudder competition at Mount Snow in Vermont. Pete was one of the league's best. He won the Most Valuable Player Award in 2010, and the game was coming easy to him.

"I had finally figured out the game," Pete recalls. "It kind of sucked that I was now twenty-six years old, but I was playing like I was twenty. I had no doubt that I would've been drafted if I were still playing at Boston College."

He was never a braggart, but he told his friends to come see him play because he was feeling really good. "I was hitting off speed and going the other way. I had always been a dead pull hitter, never off speed." The previous season, he pulled a Babe Ruth and called his own shot, and he did it with bases loaded. "I told a teammate that if I got into a count and I thought a changeup was coming, I was gonna hit it out."

Sure enough, Pete got into a 3-2 count. He paused and gripped the bat tightly. He looked over and winked at his friend and stepped back into the batter's box. The pitch came and Pete smashed it over the right field fence. "The game was easy," he says. "I was anticipating situations before they happened."

He was also a speed demon, a terror on the base paths and a vacuum in the outfield. As the season started in 2011, Pete was still making jaw-dropping catches in the outfield, such as during the game against nearby Watertown, when he snagged a fly ball as he leaped over the fence.

But suddenly, his batting average had dropped a hundred points, from .375 to .275. His bat speed was off. "I was striking out a ton and making average pitchers look like studs. I was normally one of the fastest guys in the league, but now I was lumbering around the base path, trying to get my legs moving."

He was frustrated, angry, and confused. His body was subtly, slowly, failing him, and he had no idea why.

2
WARNING SIGNS

Pete's struggles carried over with his first at bat. He was facing pitcher Jared Freni, a fireballer from the University of Massachusetts who routinely threw ninety- to ninety-five-mile-per-hour fastballs.

The Chiefs' pitcher knew Pete was struggling and the opposing ballplayers taunted him relentlessly. Fastball after fastball was pumped inside to Pete, almost daring him to snap out of his slump.

"I'm gonna catch the next one and crush it," he mumbled. His brain knew what he wanted to do, but his arms were not cooperating. The bat felt weighted in his once-powerful hands as he swung behind every pitch. *What the hell is going on?* He thought to himself. *Where is my strength?*

His father was asking the same question. "What's he doing?" John asked Nancy, as Pete fouled off another inside fastball. "He normally cleans that stuff out."

Pete needed to adjust his swing if he had any hope of connecting with the ball and getting on base. There was much on the line. The game had been a defensive struggle so far. This was game six of a seven-game series. Pete's team was up three games to two over the Chiefs and they now had the opportunity to close out the series. The Blue Sox held a one-run lead over their foes, and Pete was hoping to stretch that lead now in the fifth inning.

When the next pitch came, he jumped on the inside fastball. The fast ball missed the bat and crashed into Pete's left wrist with a loud crack! A violent jolt of pain traveled through his body. He gasped for air and his vision blurred.

"Ouch!" Nancy said to her husband.

"Jeezus," John blurted. He was surprised at the impact because Pete's hands were always quick enough to get out of the way of an inside pitch like that.

Pete had been hit by pitches before, but this one felt different. The sharp pain was overwhelming. Still, he tried to shake it off as he trotted toward first base. His parents had seen him hit by pitches too. They had also seen him take and deliver wallops in football and get crushed at center ice in hockey. No matter the impact, Pete always shook it off. This was no different, they thought. But when Pete got to first base, John could see that he was hurting badly. He was shaking his left hand and rubbing it.

For the rest of the game, Pete tried to focus on the action and his opponent, but it was impossible to do. His mind was racing as he mulled over questions that he could not answer. He had two more at bats and struck out both times. Pete's parents felt his frustration.

"My god, what's going on with him?" Nancy asked her husband. "He's just having such a bad season."

Julie watched Pete struggle as she stood on the grassy knoll near the outfield, her stomach tied in knots. *Is it nerves?* she asked herself.

Julie knew he had been in a deep slump over the past few games, so she cheered louder and louder to show him her support. "C'mon Pete, you can do it!"

Her enthusiasm caught the attention of Nancy and John. "She's a keeper," Nancy whispered to her husband.

The Blue Sox ended up losing the game on a walk-off home run. Pete's head hung low in the dugout. His father went to check on him. Pete's wrist was limp, almost hanging. John feared it was broken or that it had some serious structural damage.

"What the heck, Pete? Maybe we should just go to the hospital," his dad said.

"Don't worry about it. I'm going to go over to BC," he said. "I'll go see the trainer and they'll fix me up." Pete still had lots of friends in the Boston College baseball program and was treated like royalty around the athletic facilities. Even though he was long gone from the Chestnut Hill College, he was seen by others as the pride of the program and was always welcome on campus, even in the trainers' room.

Pete gave Julie a wave as the group of friends piled back onto the bus to continue the party at a nightclub near Boston's historical Faneuil Hall. He needed to go ice down and clean up before heading into the city to meet them. He had a sick feeling in his stomach, as this was a night he had been looking forward to for weeks.

Nancy and John made the drive back to their home in Beverly and chitchatted a bit about the game and how Pete was not acting like himself. John was worried about the injury to his son's wrist, but he didn't say much so as not to upset his wife.

"Do you think Pete is okay?" Nancy asked.

"I don't know, Nancy," John said. "I really don't know."

Their son had doubts of his own.

Later Pete arrived at the nightclub and managed to smile and put on a brave face for Julie and his friends. His girlfriend saw through the facade. While friends enjoyed a raucous time at the club, Pete stood by the bar and solemnly nursed a beer. Julie knew Pete would be a bit down because they lost, but she did not expect to see him so despondent.

Should I give him some space? She asked herself. Julie turned to Elise. "The game is really bothering him," Julie told her friend. She approached Pete at the bar and whispered in his ear. "Are you okay?" She looked into his eyes and noticed something. It was not anger over losing the game. It was fear.

"I just want to get out of here," he told her.

"Sure," she said. "No problem."

Something was truly wrong. Pete loved a good party and had been looking forward to this celebration for weeks. Julie had planned on a late night out, but by ten o'clock she and Pete were on their way back to his apartment in South Boston.

Hours later Pete's roommate Tommy Haugh brought a crew of partiers back to the apartment, but Pete just was not in the mood. He was clearly sad, and perhaps even a bit depressed, but the more Julie asked if he was okay, the more he downplayed it. She knew, though, that he was far from his usual self. Something was seriously bothering him. *But what can I tell her?* He thought to himself. *How would she understand when I don't have a clue about what's happening to me?*

3

BOSTON, 1975

"This can't be happening," Nancy D'Alfonso whispered to herself, as she sat with her mother and father in a sterile examination room at Tufts Medical Center. The attractive auburn-haired high school student should have been trying on prom dresses at this time of year, but instead she was stuck in a strange room with strange doctors trying their best to explain to her the strange tumor that had invaded and grown in her body. A mass had been found in Nancy's neck during a previous physical examination, and after several tests doctors were able to diagnose the problem. It was serious. Something was giving her severe pain and had made it difficult for her to swallow. The culprit was cancer of the thyroid.

Nancy looked over at her parents and tears began to well up in their eyes. She had always taken care of her body. She ate right and did not smoke. And she was a teenager. How could this type of cancer afflict someone so young? Her doctors explained that it was indeed a rare condition for a seventeen-year-old girl. In all cases of thyroid cancer, less than 5 percent of patients are teenagers. Nancy was now part of a special group, a group she did not want to belong to.

She was just old enough to get her driver's license and now there was a chance she would die. As a Roman Catholic, Nancy relied heavily on her faith and her strong Italian family, one that had overcome challenges to realize the American dream. Nancy's father, Ulderico D'Alfonso, the only son of immigrant parents from Chieti, Italy, was born and raised in

East Boston. His father died when Ulderico was just four years old, and his mother spoke no English. The boy relied on his four older sisters, who were both educated and industrious. One older sister, Connie, walked Ulderico to register for first grade and changed his name to Gerald, a more American-sounding name. Gerald D'Alfonso became a stellar student and earned himself a scholarship at Northeastern University to study journalism. He later landed a job with the *Salem Evening News* and relocated to the North Shore to raise a family. Her father had experienced untold hardships to provide better lives for Nancy and her three siblings, and now she would need to call on that grit and determination to face her fears.

Nancy's best option for survival was to remove her thyroid to prevent the tumor from spreading through her body. If the cancer went untreated, there was even a chance that she would die within five years. This dark reality outweighed the risks of surgery—a major blood clot in her neck or the permanent loss of her voice.

It was an easy decision for Nancy and her family. She underwent a total thyroidectomy, as surgeons made a two-inch incision across the front of her neck and successfully removed the cancerous growth. Later, as Nancy recovered in her hospital bed, she reflected on her arduous journey and discovered her inner strength. "To be faced with your own mortality as a seventeen-year-old, it was something that drove me a little more," Nancy recalls.

She was a straight A student who had missed most of the second half of her junior year. When she returned to school, she applied herself even more vigorously in the classroom and had her pick of colleges, although she applied to only one. Nancy had visited the campus of Boston College in Chestnut Hill, roughly forty miles south of Nancy's family home in Beverly. She had no friends or relatives there. It was just a school she had heard about, but she was immediately drawn to the institution for its Jesuit methods of learning and its pristine campus and beautiful gothic architecture.

Nancy applied for and received early acceptance at BC. That winter, she took a job at King's Grant, a medieval-themed restaurant and motor inn along busy Route 128 in Danvers, Massachusetts. Dressed from head to toe as a fourteenth-century maiden, Nancy waited on customers and scrubbed pots and pans along with other local teens working to raise money for college or for a night out with friends. John Frates took a job there to pay for a new car and his tuition. He lived nearby and King's Grant was just a short walk through the woods from his house. John was Irish Catholic, with a trace of Portuguese. He was tall and handsome and studied at the prestigious St. John's Prep, an all-boys school. John was naturally athletic, but he had taken a beating on the football field, so he gave up contact sports and got a part-time job cutting roast beef at the buffet station at King's Grant. At the end of each shift, John would hide slices of cooked meat under the buffet tables for the hungry wait staff to chow down in secrecy.

"It was great to meet kids from all the surrounding towns, especially the girls in the cute waitress uniforms," John recalls. One particular server caught his eye right away. John knew Nancy only slightly, having dated one of her friends. He harbored a secret crush on Nancy, and she felt the same way about him, though both wondered what they had in common with each other. He was a prep school kid, and she went to public school. He was "Boston Irish" and she was "Boston Italian." Their backgrounds appeared to be oceans apart, but their values were similar. They also shared a taste for rock music. Nancy's dad had done some entertainment reporting and editing for the *Boston Globe* and managed to score tickets to the year's hottest show at the Boston Garden. The Who was in town, and everyone was clamoring for a ticket. Nancy was going to ask an old boyfriend to go with her. That would have been easy, although her heart was not in it. She wanted to move forward in her love life, not backward, so she decided to use the tickets as an icebreaker with the handsome prep school kid.

While washing dishes at King's Grant one morning, Nancy mentioned to John that she had tickets to the show. He gushed about his love for the rock band and rattled off his favorite songs. She was impressed and asked if he would like to join her. It was a date. This they both knew, but it also lacked the pressure of having to engage in small talk over pizza. John drove Nancy into the city on the night of the concert and found parking near Boston Garden. Throngs of music fans were gathering on Causeway Street, sharing cigarettes and passing joints back and forth. The couple cut their way through the thick haze of smoke and squeezed into the Garden, standing shoulder to shoulder with thousands of Who fans, all of whom believed they were about to witness something special.

The band took the stage and lead singer Roger Daltrey powered his way through "I Can't Explain" accompanied by Pete Townsend's signature guitar riff. John and Nancy rocked out as the band segued into "Substitute." The drum beat was slightly off at first and only got worse. At the end of the song, drummer Keith Moon fell over his drum kit and passed out onstage. The crowd went wild, thinking that it was part of the group's anarchistic, hard-charging stage act. But the drummer did not get up and had to be carried backstage by some long-haired roadies.

"Keith Moon is in very bad shape," bassist John Entwistle told the crowd. "We're gonna try to work things out."

Moon's bandmates followed him offstage. Fans began to stir, and John and Nancy had no clue what was happening. Moments later The Who's front man returned to the stage. "Keith Moon has the flu," Roger Daltrey announced.

That was it. John and Nancy's first date ended after two songs. The show was cancelled, and disgruntled fans began burning trash under the Garden bleachers. Fire alarms sounded, emergency doors opened, and the concert goers poured into the cold night, chanting, "refund!" Nancy and John managed to get out safely and drove home as a light snow began to fall.

"Although we felt a few sparks on our first date, we automatically got a second chance when The Who returned for a makeup show a month later," John says. "And we haven't been apart since." John asked her on five future dates that evening, including the prom. Nancy said yes. It appeared that her cancer ordeal was far behind her now. An added bonus for Nancy was the fact that John would follow her to Boston College. He had been accepted to the University of Massachusetts but was waitlisted at BC. John recruited an uncle who was also a Jesuit priest to help him make a full-court press on the Admissions Office and was finally accepted. The two entered BC as a couple and remained that way for all four years. But they were not the type of couple that had to be with each other twenty-four hours a day. They each formed strong friendships on campus, and eventually her friends became his friends and vice versa. They survived the epic Blizzard of '78 that had paralyzed New England by treating their dorm as an Aspen ski chalet. Nancy and John took in Boston College football games and celebrated wins and forgot about losses at BC hangouts like Molly's on Harvard Avenue and Callahan's in Newton. These were carefree times for the couple and their large gang of friends, but something darker kept weighing on Nancy's mind. She kept wondering whether her cancer would come back. In December of her senior year, she had secured a job at one of the major banks in Boston and was enrolled in its commercial-lending training program. Nancy was proud of her work, but her real goal in life—her mission—was to raise a family. Because of the uncertainty of her health, Nancy wanted to start a family right away.

"I always had one important thing to be in life and that was to be a mother," she said. "So I asked John whether he was in or out." Nancy proposed to John and he accepted. He even used his student-loan proceeds to buy a ring, and the couple became formally engaged on Christmas Day. They eventually married in June 1981 at Trinity Chapel on the campus of Boston College. It was a big Italian and Irish wedding with 220 guests, mostly college friends, held at the historical restaurant Anthony's Pier 4 on Boston's waterfront. The couple's first child, a daughter named Jennifer, was born one year later. Their second child, Pete, came along on December 28, 1984, while the country was caught up in Boston College fever, following quarterback Doug Flutie's Hail Mary pass to beat the University of Miami just one month earlier. Flutie would take home the Heisman Trophy that season, while also inspiring future generations of college students entering The Heights. Nancy and John had no idea that their son would carve out an inspirational path of his own far beyond the playing fields of Boston College.

4
ONE IN TEN THOUSAND

Nancy Frates had expected to deliver her firstborn son on New Year's Eve, but she went into labor two days early at the family's Beverly home. John rushed her to the hospital, as her contractions became more frequent and more painful. What was expected to be a routine delivery was touch and go for awhile because the baby was too big for Nancy's slight frame. Finally, the newborn John Peter Frates III entered the world at eight pounds, twelve ounces. The baby was named after his father and paternal grandfather, and his proud parents first hoped to call him J. P. but later decided on Pete. The couple's initial moments of joy were soon replaced by fear and concern as the baby contracted hives and had to be placed into an incubator.

That first night in Beverly Hospital, Nancy sat in the incubator room keeping a watchful eye on her newborn son. She was exhausted and sore but refused to leave his side until a nurse strongly suggested that Nancy needed some rest to regain her strength.

"You look tired," the nurse told her. "Go get some sleep. We'll watch after him."

The nurse gave Nancy a sedative, and she returned to her hospital bed and drifted off into a deep sleep. In the middle of the night, she awoke in a daze, only to find two pediatricians standing over her bed. There was a look of grave concern on their faces.

"Nancy, I'm afraid to tell you, your baby is very sick," one doctor said. "We're not sure what's wrong but he's really sick."

Pete had blood in his stool and had lost a pound. Nancy pulled herself out of bed and rushed back to her baby's side. The child's pink body was covered with reddish welts. What doctors soon discovered, however, was that Pete had also developed a staph infection, which could be deadly. About five thousand newborns are stricken with staph infections each year and 10 percent of those cases prove to be fatal.

She grabbed the telephone and called John, who was at home caring for their daughter, Jenn. Nancy was hysterical. "He's sick, our baby is very sick," she cried. "They are calling in specialists to try something to reverse it. He may not survive the night."

John could hardly believe what he was hearing. "I just saw him a few hours ago. He was doing great." He went to the hospital, which was only a few thousand yards away from their home at the time. Doctors told John and Nancy that staph had been discovered in the nursery and that since the baby had been circumcised, the bacteria had entered his blood stream. The newborn was taken from the nursery and admitted into the pediatrics unit, where he stayed for the next six days. Nancy and John kept vigil as doctors worked to save Pete's life. The baby was injected with antibiotics twice a day until the infection finally disappeared. The couple was allowed to bring Pete home in early January. Within days the child showed no signs of illness and he bounced back quickly to become a healthy and happy baby.

He was a fighter from the start.

Nancy and John felt fortunate because Pete rarely cried and always seemed to have a smile on his curious face. He played constantly and was happily engaged with the many relatives and family friends that filled the Frates home.

From an early age Pete emerged as the leader of the pack among his classmates and friends. He always included all the neighborhood kids when they played games, especially the children that others would ignore or tease.

"He would go over the rules of each game with the rest of us to make sure we understood how to play," Jenn remembers. "He also refused to go inside. Pete would actually wet his pants while playing because he did not want to go home for anything, even for a bathroom break."

Pete also doted on his little brother, Andrew, who joined the family when Pete was three years old. The Frates had three children now, and Nancy felt that her family was complete. She had kept her ultimate promise to herself—the promise of motherhood—and she adored all of her children. But Nancy and John were not parents who overcompensated for their kids. A price had to be paid for their children's errors. It was a currency that would help build their character.

"We allowed our kids to fail. They had to fail," says Nancy. "I call it failing forward. You have to learn from your failure." Nancy would give her kids one chance—one chance to forget their homework or their lunch. She would leap into action and bring food and other materials to school but reminded the kids that they had used up their free pass. "I'm not coming next time," she told them. "You'll have to go to detention or fend for yourself. You've made a bad decision, and there are consequences for that."

This nurturing yet tough approach to parenting allowed all three children to thrive. To spend more time with her children, Nancy left her job in commercial lending and held a series of part-time jobs, from working at the kids' school to waitressing to manning phones at a call center at night. John was working in restaurant-equipment sales at the time. Both had an entrepreneurial spirit and had been discussing ways to go into business on their own. John happened to drive by a small roadside ice cream stand for sale in Beverly and knew he had found the answer. When he was out on the road meeting with restaurant owners, John saw that people in the ice cream business were the happiest people on earth. It was the late 1980s and the frozen yogurt craze had taken hold in New England and the country. John and Nancy placed a bid on the old Porter Farm Ice Cream stand, and a family business was born. They would bring in Jenn, Pete, and little Andrew and let them run around the shop while they worked. Jenn loved chocolate ice cream, and Andrew savored cookie dough, but Pete would eat only strawberry. He hated most sweets and avoided chocolates and sugary candy in favor of fruit, vegetables, and meat. He even got fruit in his Christmas stocking and Easter basket each year.

"It was frustrating at times being his sister," Jenn jokes. "He always ate healthy foods. He was also so kind to others and great at sports. We all suffered a little bit by comparison."

At work Nancy handled the bookkeeping, while John was in charge of overall maintenance. The kids grew and so did the business. John and Nancy took over another ice cream shop in a nearby mall, and they also bought a new home in Beverly.

"It's the house that frozen yogurt built," John says fondly.

When the kids were old enough, they too began serving frozen treats to customers, and the family now had enough money to afford a private education for the children. The boys would be steered toward St. John's Prep, John's alma mater, while Jenn would have to consider an all-girls high school. She was very smart and scored high grades, but she was also pragmatic. Jenn opted for public high school instead, where she knew she would flourish with or without the benefits or trappings of private education. Jenn would later attend and graduate from Boston College, as her parents had done.

At first, John and Nancy loved operating their own business, as it would allow them to spend more time with the kids—helping Jenn with homework, attending to Andrew, or watching Pete's skills develop on the ball field. But pressures of running a family-owned business continued to mount, as the heavy cost of equipment maintenance chewed into profits. The couple looked at other local ice cream shops, and they saw generational businesses, where sons and daughters were sometimes forced to keep up the family tradition. John and Nancy could not see their kids scooping ice cream and pouring frozen yogurt all their lives, so they opted to get out. A buyer came along, and the couple sold Porter Farm and the shop at the mall. With the money they earned, John and Nancy took time to reinvent themselves professionally. He began a new career as a financial advisor while she got her real estate license.

At this time, young Pete Frates was also beginning to come into his own. In fourth grade Pete had a gym teacher named Susan Stowe who taught the kids a dance curriculum. Mrs. Stowe had been teaching at the elementary school for decades and even taught Nancy when she was a child. Mrs. Stowe would demonstrate the dance routine and take the students through each step. All the children struggled to grasp the movements, but Pete would always pick it up perfectly on the first try. The exercise provided only a brief glimpse into the boy's physical and mental abilities and potential, but the teacher recognized what she saw. When she bumped into Nancy, she could not contain her excitement. "Okay, I've been waiting to say this to you," the teacher began. "I've been watching your Pete, and I think you've got a Division 1 athlete on your hands."

Mrs. Stowe had two children, who were then playing Division 1 sports in college. She studied Pete's hand-eye coordination and his foot coordination and saw something very special in the boy. "We call kids like Pete one in ten thousand," she told Nancy. That was the ratio of student athletes who competed on the elite college level.

Hearing teachers and coaches praise Pete's athleticism, dedication in the classroom, prowess, and natural leadership ability became a common refrain in the Frates family. Others also saw promise in the boy. Pete had been selected to sing a solo during a Memorial Day concert at school. Like other parents, Nancy and John had their video camera rolling to capture the moment. They were proud that Pete had the courage to stand up onstage alone in front of an auditorium full of parents, but they did not think much more of it. The next morning Nancy received a call from the director of a popular and competitive chorale group in the region who had been in the audience for the concert. The director told Nancy that she wanted Pete to join the group and would waive the normal audition process. Nancy had heard of the group, as Jenn's friends had all tried out for coveted choir spots in the past. It was an honor to be asked, but she knew Pete was focused on sports and did not want to overschedule or overwhelm the boy.

A year later John and Nancy received another random phone call from a soccer coach in the nearby town of Reading who ran a regional club team for kids fourteen and under. Pete was just old enough to play for the team, but the coach begged the Frates to let him join the squad.

"You must have the wrong parents," Nancy told the coach. "Our Pete doesn't play soccer."

"I know he doesn't play soccer but the whole coaching community is talking about him," the coach replied. "He's a natural athlete, and I can teach him soccer."

Soccer did not appeal to Pete, but he completely immersed himself in other sports, especially his three favorites: hockey, baseball, and football.

The poster of one player in particular earned prime real estate on the wall of Pete's bedroom—that of Raymond Bourque, Boston Bruins' all-world defenseman. Bourque was the Bruins' best player and also captain of the team. Bourque was not a vocal leader, at least not in public. Instead, he guided his teammates to the play-offs and two trips to the Stanley Cup Finals through a tireless work ethic and a never-ending supply of grit and determination. Whenever Pete was on the ice or firing slap shots into the upper corners of a well-worn hockey net at the end of the driveway, he emulated his sports idol. When he was not playing hockey, whacking whiffle balls, or playing tackle football in the neighborhood, he was glued to the television watching his favorite teams or following them in the box scores of the *Boston Herald* and the *Boston Globe*. He could rattle off statistics like a color analyst, reciting the goals, assists, and points for his favorite Bruins players—bruising forward Cam Neely, slick centerman Adam Oates, and, of course, Ray Bourque.

Pete loved his hometown teams, with a fierce loyalty and undying allegiance that he never lost. Every year on his birthday, Nancy would come into his room in the morning and say, "Happy Birthday, Pete."

"Thanks, Mom," he would reply. Then he would point to the Ray Bourque poster on his wall and add, "And say 'Happy Birthday' to Ray too, Mom."

Pete shared a birthday with his sports idol.

Pete wanted to play sports in high school, and his dad was nudging him to go to his alma mater, St. John's Prep. "The Prep," as it's known around the North Shore, is a sports powerhouse and well-respected academic institution. But Pete wanted to go to Beverly High School with his buddies.

Eventually Pete came around and the decision was made to follow in his dad's footsteps and attend the Prep. It was a decision that was not made easily. Pete sat at the kitchen table and mulled over his options to the point of crying. He wanted to play sports in high school and was a bit intimidated by the level of competition he would face at St. John's. Finally, his sister, Jenn, walked in from cross-country practice and cuffed her little brother in the back of the head, as only she could.

"What's the matter with you?" she asked. "If I had had the chance to go to the Prep, don't you think I'd be there?"

Despite early reservations, he settled in nicely at St. John's. It was also a pivotal decision, because it was freshman year when he met who would become his lifelong best friend, Tommy Haugh. Tommy was a quiet kid. Their mothers grew up together in Beverly, and it was not long before the boys were inseparable. They formed a brotherhood, and Tommy grew to become the rock in Pete's life that he could always count on, no matter where he went or what was happening.

Pete sprouted several inches freshman year and started bulking up a bit. He was already a well-known athlete, but now that he was gaining size he was catching the attention of the coaches and the upper classmen, not only because of his athletic prowess, but also because of his work ethic. Like his hero Ray Bourque, he was determined to never be outworked by anyone. And it was noticed.

In his first year Pete went out for the freshman hockey team. At St. John's, hockey is a marquee sport with a rich history of success, in a state known for elite prep and private schools that consistently feed Division 1 hockey programs and the National Hockey League. Ninety kids tried out for the freshman hockey team that year, and the two-week tryout was grueling.

On the night of final cuts, parents sat waiting nervously for news in the lobby of the Ristuccia Arena in nearby Wilmington. The rink is St. John's home ice but also served for years as the practice facility for the Boston Bruins. As parents wrought their hands, waiting for their sons to emerge from the locker room, players streamed out one by one, some smiling and happy, and others dejected, having been cut from the squad.

It was a tense wait, but when Pete came out, he was smiling and was followed by the coach. "I made it. I made it," Pete proudly told his parents. Nancy and John were elated.

Coach John Holden was equally satisfied with the outcome, telling the family, "Not only do I have my defenseman; I also have my captain."

Pete remained captain of the hockey team and later captained the baseball team during his senior year at St. John's.

As Pete starred on the ice and the ball fields, that freshman year was a gloriously innocent time at the Frates household. It was marked by sleepovers, ice hockey until dark on the small pond down the street, more pizza nights than you could count, and the din of constant laughter filling the family's homey two-story colonial. The house served as headquarters for the Prep kids; the door was always open, and it was not uncommon for there to be seven or eight kids sleeping over on a Friday night.

Pete's leadership skills followed him from sports and into the classroom. Pete was struggling in one of his classes, advanced-placement biology, and was worried about an upcoming parent-teacher conference with the instructor. He tried to prepare Nancy and John for what would most likely be a painful conversation with the teacher. "I don't know why they put me in Level 1 Bio," he told his parents.

They entered the laboratory classroom and took a seat across from the teacher and waited. After a long pause the instructor pointed firmly at Nancy.

"You know he has it, you know that, right?" the teacher asked. "He has *it.*"

The *it* that the teacher was referring to was a combination of compassion for others, intellectual curiosity, and leadership. Pete's personality could be the focus of a lab experiment all its own. He personified the age-old question—are leaders born or are they made?

Most close observers looked at Pete as a born leader. Leadership scholars believe that those with the natural ability to lead others have several common innate traits, such as inclusiveness, sympathy, generosity of spirit, team orientation, and charisma. Pete had exhibited all these qualities from a very early age. The question was, how would these rare qualities best serve others? The Frates family thought they would find the answer in sports, but ultimately he would prove them wrong.

5

FEARLESS

A car pulled up to the Kowalik family home in Marblehead and out stepped two academic types, carrying folders and a toy robot. They rang the doorbell and Joe Kowalik answered and ushered them inside. They could hear the delightful sound of a toddler playing in a nearby room. The researchers sat down at the kitchen table with the child's father and further explained what they had discussed on the phone.

At only fourteen months old, Joe's daughter, Julie, had been selected to participate in a scientific study to analyze how young children responded to fear. The scientists from Harvard University stressed that Joe's daughter would not be in any danger or physical pain during the exercises and that she would not hold any memories of the sessions.

Satisfied, Joe got up from the table and retrieved his daughter from her bedroom. The little girl bounced into the kitchen and smiled at the strangers. Julie Kowalik was not shy; this the researchers found out right away. The scientists spoke to the girl softly and gained her trust. It helped that Julie's dad was in the room. They asked her father if they could place the child alone in a room with a big toy robot and study her reaction. The researchers had done this experiment with other toddlers, and most were frightened by the battery-operated robot's awkward movements. As the robot was turned on and began to move forward and backward in the little girl's bedroom, Julie studied it for a moment and then walked over, curled her tiny hand into a fist, and smashed the robot over its head. The scientists were astounded at the lack of fear in young Julie Kowalik. They started coming to the family home more often and conducted more tests. Julie always exceeded their expectations and was found to have extremely low levels of natural fear.

Results from the study later appeared in *Newsweek*, where the reporter referenced Julie. "She may be less than 3 feet tall, but Julie is not easily intimidated. When an unfamiliar woman enters the room, the 14-month-old waddles over to investigate," the reporter wrote. "She's delighted when the stranger lets a three-foot-tall battery-operated robot out of the closet and is unfazed when a researcher starts churning a lottery cage with colorful balls. These are the Ethel Mermans of the world." *The fearless ones.*

The researchers would continue to track Julie and other test subjects throughout the children's adolescence, their teenaged years, and into adulthood. At age twenty-one, she was given a full CAT scan for six hours to monitor her neurological development. The result was consistent with all the experiments up to that point. Julie Kowalik was considered to be fearless.

She was also academically gifted, more so than her future boyfriend Pete Frates. Julie's dad was an executive with Polaroid who had played both baseball and football while studying engineering at Cornell University. Joe Kowalik went on to earn a master's degree at Harvard before settling down with his love, Mary Kate (Finn), in Marblehead.

Julie's mom, Mary Kate, known simply as Kate to her family and friends, grew up in Marblehead with four siblings. A tight-knit Irish family, the Finns all stuck around Marblehead and remain very close today. Kate got her law degree from Suffolk University Law School but became a homemaker once she had the couple's first child, a boy they named Joseph, after his father. On January 11, 1990—Kate's birthday—she received the greatest birthday gift of her life: a beautiful baby girl they named Julie.

The family lived at 60 Seaview Avenue in Marblehead, a picturesque seaside neighborhood on Preston Beach near the Swampscott town line. Kate's sisters lived right up the street, and Julie's two cousins, Amy and Maddy, were her constant playmates and became her best friends growing up. They were more like sisters than cousins, as the Finn family spent most of its social time together, whether it was at family parties, sun-filled days at the beach, or up at Kezar Lake in New Hampshire. It was an idyllic childhood for Julie and her brother. Joe and Kate were always there for the kids' sports games. Mom picked her and Joseph up from school every day. The holidays were like a real-life Norman Rockwell painting.

They belonged to the Beach Club in Swampscott, and Julie spent most of her childhood summers there, swimming, playing beach games, eating ice cream, and reveling in the beauty of the Atlantic Ocean. She was on the swim team at the beach club and stayed there most nights until long after dark—usually as late as nine o'clock.

When Julie was in sixth grade, the whole extended family took a trip to Ireland. It was just after the terror attacks of September 11, 2001, and some in the family were nervous about flying, especially Julie's grandfather, who hated to fly anyway. But they all made it over and spent an incredible week there, including celebrating Thanksgiving in Galway. Julie, Maddy, and Amy were just tweens and had the time of their lives, walking the cobblestone streets of Galway, visiting the lush ocean cliffs, and spending time with their entire family. They rented out a whole floor of a local restaurant and had a special Thanksgiving dinner. It is one of Julie's fondest memories, as it was the last trip she ever took with her grandparents, who have since passed away.

Another family-bonding trip occurred during Julie's sophomore year of high school, when the Kowaliks went to Italy and rented villas in Chianti. Julie was just fifteen years old, and she learned to drive on that trip, navigating the winding streets of Italy with her family in their rented station wagon. The experience inspired Julie to study abroad in Florence when she got to Boston College a few years later.

In high school Julie was very popular, got straight As, and was on the soccer and basketball teams. She and her group of friends were not angels, but they stayed out of trouble, for the most part. High school was a cherished experience for Julie, filled with sports, parties, and sleepovers every weekend. She was a typical boy-crazy teenage girl, and she had a couple of semiserious boyfriends in high school. Many people in Marblehead have boats, so the teenagers would often sneak onto someone's parents' boat and drink. Once, when she was a freshman, Julie snuck out with a group of kids onto someone's boat at the yacht club. They took a joyride, but when they pulled back into the dock, Julie's mom was standing there, waiting for her. The stunt earned her a week of being grounded, and Joe and Kate made her paint a fence at the house.

—

Joe Kowalik's approach to parenting was similar to John and Nancy Frates: he nurtured his children, but if they screwed up, they had to pay the price. Despite these tough-love tactics, Julie considered herself to be one of the fortunate ones. She was beautiful and smart, and she lived a comfortable life devoid of conflict or struggle. If she ever faced a serious dilemma in life, how would she respond? Julie was not a girl who was battle tested, but she had one unique trait that would help her weather the coming storm. She was fearless.

6
NEW HEIGHTS

In late January 1999 Boston College announced the hiring of its new head baseball coach, Pete Hughes. For a college sports program that was thriving in the Big East at the time, it was an inauspicious announcement. But for Pete Frates, it was life changing.

Baseball was largely an afterthought at BC, which had a dominant hockey program and football and basketball teams that competed in the nation's best conferences and were regularly featured on national television. The football team, led by future NFL quarterback and ESPN analyst Tim Hasselbeck, had just come off another impressive season, going 8–4 in the Big East under Coach Tom O'Brien. Hasselbeck, son of New England Patriots tight end Don Hasselbeck and brother of NFL star Matt Hasselbeck, led the Eagles to the Insight.com Bowl, where they lost to the University of Colorado.

The basketball team, perennial contenders for the Big East crown and occasional invitees to the NCAA tourney, was rebuilding under head coach Al Skinner, while the hockey team was its usual juggernaut, landing in the 1999 Frozen Four under Jerry York, considered by many to be the best college coach in the country. All three programs were regularly shipping players to the pro ranks throughout the 1990s, including the Hasselbecks; quarterback Glenn Foley; All-Pro linemen Tom Nalen, Damian Woody, and Pete Kendall; NBA players Dana Barros, Billy Curley, and Howard

Eisley; and NHL stars Brian Leetch, Bill Guerin, Brooks Orpik, and Kevin Stevens.

The baseball program, though, had not been able to climb out of the Big East cellar. The Eagles had only two winning seasons in the 1990s and none since 1993. They had averaged just thirteen wins a year over the three decades before Hughes's arrival.

Hughes grew up in Brockton, Massachusetts, a tough, blue-collar city of a hundred thousand just south of Boston. Hailing from a large Irish American family, his brother played football for Brockton High School, the state's largest public high school and a gridiron powerhouse in the 1970s, 1980s, and 1990s. He chose instead to attend Boston College High School, an all-boys Catholic school in the Dorchester section of Boston. There he was a standout infielder for the Eagles and quarterbacked the football team, earning Catholic Conference MVP honors in baseball and a slot in the Shriner's All-Star Game for his QB play. Hughes also earned a scholarship to Davidson College in North Carolina, where he was the starting quarterback for three seasons and a standout third baseman who for years held the school record for doubles.

Upon his graduation from Davidson, Hughes became an assistant football coach at Hamilton College in upstate New York, earning just $3,000 and living in a one-bedroom apartment above a frat house, which he fondly recalls as a "cell." The young coach endured the squalor to follow his dream of becoming a college coach. Only it wasn't football where he was destined to make his mark.

After the short-lived Hamilton job, he landed a position as assistant baseball coach at Northeastern University in Boston, where he learned the ropes for a few seasons. In 1997 he was named head coach at Division 3 Trinity University in Texas, where he posted a 52–30 record over two seasons. He also got married to his college sweetheart, Debby.

Boston College's struggling program needed some fresh blood, and Hughes, with his Boston roots, deep baseball knowledge, and overall drive to win, was just what the school was looking for to give the team a much-needed morale boost. Baseball was a nearly invisible fourth out of the major sports on campus, and it had become accepted that fielding a nationally competitive team in a cold-weather city like Boston, where it snowed or was cold half the year, was not realistic. Hughes was determined to change that.

"This year is going to be a challenge for our team," Hughes said at his introductory press conference. "We are going to have to outcompete people every day."

He took over for beloved but struggling coach Richard "Moe" Maloney, who had a ten-year record of 191-209-4. Maloney's teams won three titles in the Baseball Beanpot, an annual round-robin tourney held at Fenway Park between BC, Harvard, Northeastern, and the University of Massachusetts for bragging rights in the city. But Maloney had mustered only three winning seasons.

Hughes put his own stamp on the program, and the results were immediate. He steered the 1999 squad to a 26–21 record in his first year, which at the time was the most wins in school history. Fourteen players batted over .300, which gave the Eagles a second-in-the-nation team batting average of .354. His second year was even better, as the squad went 35–20 and made its second-ever Big East Tournament. In 2002 the Eagles went 30–25, came in third in the Big East, and again made the conference tourney. The program was getting better and becoming more competitive, just as Pete was entering his senior year in high school and setting his sights on The Heights for his collegiate baseball career.

Pete Hughes first met Pete during his junior year at St. John's Prep, when he attended a baseball camp the new BC coach was running in Danvers, Massachusetts. There were 120 college hopefuls at the camp, about 10 of whom Hughes was considering as recruits. Pete was not on Hughes's radar. In fact, the coach had no idea who he was.

But Pete was determined to make an impression. On the first day of camp, he strode up to the coach and told him, point-blank, "I want to play baseball at Boston College."

Hughes was taken aback, but he did not see Pete's statement as cocky or pushy. He saw it as quietly confident and resolved. Hughes looked into Pete's background and saw that his parents were both BC alums. He also looked into Pete's playing career and saw that he was only a part-time player his junior season. If the young man could not crack the starting lineup for his high school team, what were the chances that he would play at an emerging D-1 program like Boston College? Hughes and his fellow college coaches generally recruited their players based on their junior seasons in high school. By their senior season, most players have already committed and slots are full at most colleges.

But Pete was persistent and always made himself noticed at the camp. He ran hardest in the running drills. He took extra batting and fielding practice. He was always first in line when the coaches called the players over for drills. Hughes had no choice but to lock in on Pete, because the player was relentless and put himself on his radar every chance he got. And it made an impression.

Pete's senior year at St. John's Prep was a mixture of euphoric highs and depressing lows. He started at safety on a football team stacked with Division 1 and even pro-level talent, including running back and future New York Giants player Jonathan Goff; linebacker Nick Borseti, who played at the University of Notre Dame; receiver Matt Antonelli, who would go on to play pro baseball for six seasons; tight end Jon Loyte, who played at Vanderbilt University and Boston College; and linebacker Mike Pitt, who played at Northeastern University. The Prep football teams in the early 2000s were some of the best in the school's storied history, and Pete was honored to be a part of the tradition.

The 2001 team went 11–1, only to lose in the play-offs to Everett. The 2002 squad was looking for revenge and went undefeated on its way to the Division 1 Eastern Massachusetts Super Bowl against Everett. Ten thousand rabid fans from St. John's and Everett packed into Rocky Marciano Stadium in Brockton to watch the state's two top teams clash once again in a winner-take-all battle.

Before the game Pete, a captain and one of the team's most vocal leaders, was cranking heavy metal music and psyching up his teammates. He was sure his squad was going to outplay Everett and avenge the previous year's crushing play-off loss.

Tied at seven in the third quarter, the Eagles drove down the field on a methodical, sixteen-play drive that ate up nearly eight minutes of the third quarter. The drive stalled at the Everett seven-yard line on fourth down, leaving Prep coach Jim O'Leary with a decision: kick a field goal or go for the touchdown. He opted for the latter. Quarterback Johnny McCarthy, who had thrown just two interceptions all season, fired a pass toward the end zone, but Everett defensive back Frank Nuzzo read the play perfectly, stepped in front of the pass, and snatched it at the three-yard line, running it back ninety-seven yards for a touchdown to put his team up 13–7. Nuzzo's father, Frank Sr., had pulled off a similar miracle play in 1972, running back an interception a hundred yards for a touchdown to beat undefeated Medford for the Greater Boston League title.

St. John's had one final chance and drove the ball down from its own seven-yard line to the Everett 15. Running back Steven Van Note, who went on to play for Dartmouth College, took a handoff on second-and-eight and burst through a hole in the line. He was headed for the end zone with nothing but green grass in front of him when Everett sophomore Richard Thomas leaped at him and punched the ball loose. The ball rolled into the end zone, bounced off a Prep player and was recovered by Everett, sealing the upset.

Pete was devastated by the heartbreaking, loss but he did his best to learn from the defeat. He stewed about it for several days, self-analyzing what more, if anything, he could have done to have changed the outcome. He hated to lose, but if such a loss could also be a learning experience, something positive could be gained and applied to his next challenge.

He soon swapped his cleats for ice skates and focused on hockey season—his favorite sport. St. John's Prep went 11-5-2 and made the field for the Division 1 Super Eight Tournament—the state's most elite high school tournament. Pete was captain and one of the team's starting defensemen, and he was known for his highly physical style of play. Pete's team played its first tournament game against Belmont High School and lost 5–2, bumping them out of the Super Eight and back into the Division 1 State Championship field, where they came up short in the semifinals.

Pete progressed on to baseball season and looked to the diamond for some relief from the football and hockey heartbreakers. The baseball team was also loaded and a preseason favorite to win the state title.

They repeated as Catholic Conference champions but fell short in the state tournament, losing to top-seeded Peabody, 2–1, in the semifinals. Pete, who captained the team, was named a Catholic Conference all-star. He had gone from part-time player to conference all-star in just one year and hoped that college recruiters would take notice. Pete had an official recruitment visit at Middlebury College in Vermont over Winter Break. He asked his best friend, Tommy Haugh, to tag along.

"Dude, how am I supposed to come with you?" Tommy asked him.

"Just come. I want my friend's opinion," Pete replied.

The buddies drove up to Middlebury in Pete's mother's car and, upon meeting the coach, Pete told him that Tommy was his best friend and was helping him make the decision. He also asked the coach for some meal passes for Tommy.

Williams College was next. The football coach there was Dick Farley from Danvers, close to Beverly. During a campus visit, Coach Farley was frank with Pete. "I'm going to be honest, your high school team could probably beat our team right now," the coach said. Farley confessed that St. John's plays before more fans on Thanksgiving than attend Williams' games all season. It was not exactly the lure Pete was looking for.

He was ultimately offered a full scholarship to Iona College in New York for football, a football and hockey scholarship to Fairfield University in Connecticut, packages for Williams and Middlebury, and a full scholarship to play baseball at the University of Vermont. But Boston College, the one school he desperately wanted to attend, was still just out of reach.

Pete stayed in touch with Coach Hughes, routinely peppering him with phone calls and e-mails, checking in to see if Hughes was going to find a slot for him. Friends of the Frates who knew Hughes put in calls on Pete's behalf. Clearly, there was a campaign to win Hughes over, but the coach was not convinced. He did not have any more scholarships to offer, as the school had only three baseball scholarships at the time. And even if he could get Pete in, he was not sure Pete was good enough to compete at the Division 1 level.

Pete was what Hughes calls a "classic Northeast three-sport star." He had incredible athleticism to play football, hockey, and baseball, but his baseball skills were slow to develop because he concentrated so much on the other sports. Athletes in warmer climates honed their baseball skills by playing year-round, which is why the best players often hail from states where shoveling snow is not part of the training regimen.

But Hughes saw a lot of qualities in Pete that he knew would be an asset to his team: persistence, optimism, dedication. Pete never gave up and he never gave in. He also bombarded Hughes with video highlights of his play. Normally, those are furnished by a high school coach, but Pete was not leaving anything to chance. Coach Hughes respected the initiative.

It showed tremendous drive. Pete was always the highest-energy player at Hughes's camps. He was tough. He was vocal but not a loudmouth. He had all the intangibles. So why was Hughes holding back?

When the weeks on the calendar passed, and there was still no word from BC, Pete decided that the University of Vermont was his best option. He even put a UVM sticker on the Ford truck he drove himself and Andrew to school in every day.

High school graduation came in June, and it was a foregone conclusion that Pete was going to the University of Vermont and that Boston College just was not in the cards. Pete got himself excited about the idea of moving to Burlington, and he admired the history of the baseball program at UVM. For one, the team played in one of the oldest stadiums in the country, a classic New England ball yard that was built in 1906.

On high school graduation day, the Frates family traveled to the Prep's Danvers campus and took their seats. After a few minutes an admissions counselor from the school approached the family and told them they were in the wrong seats. Because John was also an alumni, the Frates were considered a "legacy" family and were given the honor of sitting in a special section up front. The admissions counselor had something else to say. The words would change Pete's life.

"Pete, I just heard from a friend who runs the Admissions Office at BC, and he said, 'Pete's in,'" the counselor told the family.

The family was elated. Nancy and John embraced and hugged their son as tightly as they had in years. The dream of their oldest son attending their alma mater was finally coming true. Pete was excited but took the news very casually, almost professionally. It was almost as though he had expected it. To Pete, it felt like it was predetermined and that Boston College was his destiny.

7

BIRDBALL

Arriving at Boston College in the fall of 2003, Pete was overjoyed and had a swagger, not only because he had achieved his goal of attending his parents' alma mater, but because he was in peak physical condition and playing some of his best baseball.

Coach Hughes had finally decided to take a flyer on the tough and determined kid from Beverly. Hughes appreciated Pete's moxie, even though Pete had inundated him with video clips of his schoolboy baseball highlights to the point of annoyance.

"Even if he doesn't play one inning for me, he'll still make everybody better," Hughes told his assistants.

Boston College in the late 1990s was in the midst of a building boom, as it was fast becoming one of the top-tier schools in the country. Established by Jesuit priests in 1863, the liberal arts college was originally founded as a commuter school for young men living in Boston. The school nearly closed in the early 1970s due to fiscal problems that plunged the college $6 million into debt, and it was close to being acquired by Harvard University.

But the sinking academic ship was righted by Boston College president J. Donald Monan, a Jesuit priest who led the school out of the financial morass with the assistance of a newly restructured board of trustees. The board added members of the business community to bring some outside experience and ideas to the Jesuits in charge at the time. It was the same model that was used to rescue the University of Notre Dame when that school ran into similar problems.

The result was a stronger, more focused Boston College that grew fast. Majors were added, the endowments started to flourish, and the sports programs, which provided New England with its only Division 1 action, began to excel. Today, BC is recognized as one of the top thirty colleges in the country.

When Pete landed at Boston College, winning was a way of life in the three major sports programs. The hockey program had always been elite. The squad won the national championship in 1949, had made the NCAA tournament thirty-five times, and had been in the final "Frozen Four" semifinals a record twenty-five times. The hockey team owned the Hockey East, along with its Commonwealth Avenue archrival Terriers at Boston University, and was stacked with future NHL players, including Brian Boyle, brothers Ben and Patrick Eaves, Stephen Gionta, Andrew Alberts, Peter Harrold, and Ryan Shannon. Coach Jerry York's squad had won the national championship two years earlier and went on to have a very successful 2003–04 season, winning the Beanpot and the Hockey East en route to yet another Frozen Four appearance.

The football team was similarly flush with future NFL players, including Jeremy Trueblood, Jamie Silva, Chris Snee, and Mathias Kiwanuka. Coach Tom O'Brien's team had a strong running attack, led by running back Derrick Knight, who had a brief NFL career and went 8–5, including a stunning road win over QB Marcus Vick and his twelfth-ranked Virginia Tech Hokies. The Eagles lost in the San Francisco Bowl to Colorado State on New Year's Eve that season.

The basketball team, led by future pros Craig Smith and Jared Dudley, went 23–9 and was a sixth seed in the NCAA national tournament. The Eagles beat the University of Utah 58–51 in the first round but lost a 57–54 heartbreaker in the second to Georgia Tech.

Pete immersed himself in the sports culture at Boston College, followed all the teams with great passion and pride, and was a regular at games at The Heights. He was also a gym rat who constantly worked out, right alongside all the future professionals around him, impressing many with his strength and stamina. At six feet, two inches, and 215 pounds, even as a freshman Pete was one of the bigger guys on the baseball squad and certainly was one of the strongest and fastest.

While he was there to study communications and history and to play baseball, Pete still thought of himself as a classic Northeast three-sport athlete and wondered if he could play football and hockey. Many of his friends still say he likely could have walked on to the football team. Others say he never really got over his love of hockey—which his parents insist was always his favorite.

"Damn, I wish I was on the hockey team," Pete would tell his baseball friends during freshman year.

He was a big, strong, forceful guy with a long history on the ice and gridiron, and it was difficult for him to get the more physical contact sports out of his system. As he adjusted to BC and the baseball regimen, his teammates constantly busted his chops, ribbing him about wishing he was a hockey player.

The baseball team, under Coach Hughes, was making strides every year. Perennially .500 or under for years before his arrival, Hughes had the Eagles soaring. He led the team to its first winning season in six seasons in his first year, posting a 26–21 record in 1999, which was the most wins in Boston College history at the time. He posted winning seasons the next four years and went 33–21 the year before Pete landed at The Heights.

One of the first friends he made on campus was Ryne Reynoso, a right-fielder/pitcher from Hailey, Idaho, a tiny town near the Sun Valley ski resort. Reynoso, like Pete, was recruited by Hughes, but his position on the team was not very secure and was entirely dependent on how he developed as a player.

There were seven players in the 2003–04 freshmen class, but it was Pete who stood out most to Ryne. The first time they met, Pete had his beloved Red Sox cap on. He was tanned and physically imposing. He also had an air of quiet confidence.

Oh damn, this dude looks like he can play some baseball, Ryne said to himself. *This is the guy I gotta beat.*

Although they were both outfielders competing for playing time, Pete and Ryne quickly started hanging out and endured those early days of the Hughes tough training camps together. The rigorous program included team workouts, personal fitness regimens, and regular team meetings. Hughes was hard on his players, as he knew the only way Boston College could compete was to outwork their rival schools in the Big East and, later, the Atlantic Coast Conference. This was big-time college baseball, and Coach Hughes was not interested in cellar dwelling. He had won everywhere he had coached and planned on keeping it that way.

Hughes ran the players hard and was an intimidating presence on the field. With dark hair, a strong jaw, and a muscular, athletic frame, Hughes looked like he could jump on the field and play. He was stern and always had his bullshit detector on high alert. He had a dry sense of humor, and when players talked to him, they knew immediately they were dealing with a tough coach who had been through enough battles to know what leads to wins and losses.

It did not take Pete and Ryne long to get on Coach Hughes's bad side, however. One night during their first semester, before they had even played an inning, the two pals were caught partying in their dorm on upper campus with several other underage athletes and female students. The group was playing beer pong, cranking tunes, and generally raising hell, in blatant violation of the residence hall's quiet hours. The police arrived, and it was Pete and Ryne who were fingered as the ringleaders.

The cops took them into custody and drove them off in the back of a police cruiser. They were shuttled to St. Elizabeth's Hospital, a small medical center near campus where drunken students are often taken to sleep off binges, have their stomachs pumped, or get patched up from boozy injuries. The police officers kept telling Pete and Ryne they were drunk, so they needed to be checked out by the doctors. Apparently, it was a "scared straight" move by the cops, who did not want to charge them criminally but wanted to teach them a lesson. They were held at the hospital for several hours, driven back to the dorm, and released without any charges. When they got back to campus, about a half hour later, a fire alarm sounded, ending any hopes of sleep that night.

Lack of sleep was the least of their worries, however, as a police report detailing the drunken antics made it to Coach Hughes's desk, unbeknownst to the two freshmen. Hughes called them into his office two days later. He was fuming. "You two are barely even good enough to play at this school. You're really pushing it," Hughes said sternly, pointing his finger at them. "I should kick you guys off the team."

It was just before Winter Break, and Hughes made no commitment that their positions on the team were safe, instead leaving them to twist in the wind over the month-long vacation. Plus, their parents were notified, which made for a miserable first college break for Pete. John and Nancy were not happy that their son had gotten busted for underage drinking in his first semester, especially after the difficulty he had getting into the school in the first place.

When they got back from break, Hughes called them back in and told them they would have to show him they were committed to the team and school and were not just there to party. "If you want it, prove it," he said.

Pete took those words to heart. He worked extra hard after that setback and earned a roster spot on the traveling squad, while Ryne did not. As a freshman, Pete appeared in twelve games and was used mostly as a utility player and pinch hitter/runner. He had his first college at bat against Valparaiso on March 4, 2004. He scored his first run on April 25 in a thrilling 7–6 extra-inning win over the University of Connecticut. He also scored another run in a 12–5 victory over Seton Hall on May 22 and was inserted into the lineup to play left field in a Big East tournament victory over the University of Pittsburgh.

As the months went by, Pete grew into a leadership role for Coach Hughes and his Eagles. Boston College was not an easy place to play college baseball. The field doubled as a parking lot for tailgating for football games. After games Hughes would have his players walk the field, picking up bottles, charcoal, and trash. Many of the players thought it was beneath them, but Pete understood the lesson and always showed up with a smile. He led the cleanup crew, loud and proud, and made it fun. His positivity was infectious. He inspired his teammates and helped them see that cleaning up the field was a privilege and a point of pride, not a punishment.

Still, Pete was a college student, and college students like to have fun. His shenanigans freshman year were not restricted to Boston College. He and his former St. John's Prep football teammate Mike Pitt, a six-foot, four-inch redhead lineman for Northeastern University, decided one weekend to go visit their pal Tommy Haugh at Bentley College, a small private school located about nine miles west of Boston in Waltham. It was 2004 and Pete's beloved New England Patriots were vying for their second Super Bowl of the Tom Brady era.

Pete and Mike arrived at Tommy's room at Slade Hall, a dry freshman residence hall, with a bottle of 151-proof rum and were ready to let loose. The bottle was done by halftime and the boys were well lubricated, so much so that they barely paid attention to Janet Jackson's infamous "wardrobe malfunction" with Justin Timberlake during the halftime show at Reliant Stadium in Houston.

The Patriots defeated the Carolina Panthers 32–29 on a game-winning field goal with four seconds left by kicker Adam Vinatieri that followed yet another fourth quarter drive by Brady. Like the rest of Boston, the Bentley campus erupted upon the final tick of the clock that sealed the heart-stopping win and added to Brady's legacy. Pete, Tommy, and Mike ran with a rabid pack of students toward the Bentley quad, where a wild celebration broke out. Pete, wearing a cowboy hat, was a ringleader in the chaos, which included fireworks being set off.

At some point Pitt got into a fistfight that culminated with him tackling a kid in the hallway. He ran for cover when police showed up but was found hiding in a closet in the basement of a residence hall and was taken into custody. Pete evaded capture and took a cab back to Boston College. Tommy Haugh had passed out in the bathroom. The next day, as Tommy shook the cobwebs out of his aching head, campus police showed up at his room.

"Are Mike Pitt and Pete Frates friends of yours?" the cop asked.

"Yeah," Tommy said.

"Are you aware of their actions last night?" the officer said.

"Not really," Tommy said, answering honestly, as he was passed out during the height of the mayhem.

"They won't be welcome back here on the Bentley campus," Tommy was informed.

A few days later Pete received a letter in the mail, informing him he was banned from the Bentley College campus for life. So when his brother, Andrew, decided to go to Bentley the following year, Pete was concerned that he would never be able to go visit him. Pete avoided the campus for a couple of years but finally decided during his senior year that he would pay a visit. Andrew was always visiting him at BC, and Pete figured it was only fair that he experienced his brother's school with him.

"Do you think they'll know I'm your brother?" Pete asked Andrew as they discussed whether he should visit.

"It's fine, dude. Don't sweat it," Andrew assured Pete.

They decided Pete would pick Andrew up at his dorm and go to an off-campus party. When Pete pulled up in his car, he was slouched down low and had his hat pulled down.

"Hurry up and get in!" Pete shouted, as though they were pulling off a bank heist. The mission was successful, but to this day Pete is technically banned from the campus.

———

As a sophomore, Pete and some college friends became early practitioners of a social-media networking service called Facebook. The website was launched by a group of Harvard University students led by Mark Zuckerberg. Originally, the site was limited to Harvard students but expanded to other schools, including Boston College. Zuckerberg's initial goal was to set up an online data bank that allowed guys to rate and rank the beauty of campus coeds. It then transformed into a social-media café where students could chat and make plans to hit the local bars and nightclubs. Pete used the site regularly for a while but eventually got bored with it.

"I'm so done with FB," he told his dad, who discovered the site for himself when it expanded beyond a students-only portal.

As more people, young and old, began creating Facebook profiles to share photos and thoughts with friends and family, Pete was already riding the next social-media waves of Twitter and Instagram. He had no idea at the time how these social-media platforms would change his life and the lives of millions of others around the world.

When he was not fiddling with social-media applications, Pete's primary focus remained baseball. On the road with his teammates, he was like a little kid at summer camp. He was hyper and always pumped up to travel with his friends and do what he loved most: play ball. His energy was a welcome asset, but sometimes he would take it too far, and Coach

Hughes had to calm him down. Whether it was on the bus, in pregame warm-ups, practice, or the dugout, if there was a ruckus going on, nine times out of ten Pete was involved. But all it would take would be a pointed "calm down" from the coach, and Pete would step right back in line.

Despite Pete's penchant for excitement, Hughes knew he had a true locker room leader in Pete, and he would always have him host new recruits when they came on campus visits. Pete set the tone for the team, knew what Hughes expected, and could give recruits a very realistic sense of what it meant to play baseball at Boston College.

During his sophomore year, Pete played in thirty-two games, including eight starts in left field and one start at designated hitter. He did not have a great year at the plate, batting just .130 in forty-six at bats, but he had some high points. He scored six runs and had four RBIs, stole three bases in four attempts, and smacked a two-run, game-winning home run to beat Seton Hall University and secure a three-game series sweep.

Pete also made it a habit of collecting friends. His social circle was not small. Students were drawn to him because of his welcoming attitude. Joseph Ayers was one of many players that Pete took under his wing. Ayers hailed from Alaska and had transferred from Stanford University to Boston College for a better chance at a starting position on the baseball team. The transition was difficult for Ayers. It was a new school, new players, and a part of the country he had never visited before. He felt like a freshman again as he looked for ways to fit in. Pete was one of the first guys he met on campus.

"It was like, boom, best friends," Ayers recalls. "From that moment, we hit together, ate together in the cafeteria, lifted together. He introduced me to everyone he knew, which was about 95 percent of the Boston College campus."

In Pete's junior year he really came into his own on the field, playing in all fifty-three games and starting forty-five in center field. He hit .244 for the season in 160 appearances, stole a team-high nineteen bases, shared the team lead in home runs with his friend Ryne Reynoso with five, and had a nine-game hitting streak. He also went 2-for-2 and swiped two bases in a 3–2 victory over ninth-ranked Clemson University. He batted .400-plus in series victories over fifth-ranked Georgia Tech and Maryland and led the team in putouts for the year with 121.

Hughes recalled an early-season game at Virginia Tech during Pete's junior year when it was snowing in Blacksburg, Virginia. It was thirty degrees, the wind was howling, and it was snowing hard as they arrived at the ball field. Before anyone had a chance to complain, Pete hopped out of the bus with a spring in his step, wearing his uniform without any sleeves underneath, making a beeline for the snowy infield. The Virginia Tech players did not take batting practice because of the weather, but Pete sure did. He rallied his teammates, telling them, "All right, boys. It's over. They don't want to even take BP outside. It's all over. Let's go."

Boston College swept Virginia Tech that weekend, marking the team's first-ever series sweep in the powerful Atlantic Coast Conference, which BC had just joined.

That season also brought Pete's greatest baseball moment, which came at his beloved Fenway Park, the cathedral of baseball. Fenway truly was a field of dreams for Pete and his teammates. Babe Ruth had played on this field, as did Ted Williams and Carl Yastrzemski, along with more recent greats, including Pedro Martinez and David "Big Papi" Ortiz. Pete was eager to make his own mark on the legendary ball field. Boston College was playing in the annual Beanpot Tournament, pitting the city's collegiate rivals against one another. The Beanpot was a carryover from the popular collegiate hockey tournament played every year at the Boston Garden. Baseball's version drew a much smaller crowd, but for Pete it was the big stage. The Eagles fought their way to the championship game against Harvard University. Boston College had trounced the Crimson during their previous encounter that season, and Pete was eager to give BC fans a repeat performance.

John, Nancy, and his brother, Andrew, purchased their five-dollar tickets and took their seats in the iconic ball park. The Eagles jumped out to an early lead and never looked back. Pete led the way, getting a base hit each time he stepped up to the plate. His family cheered wildly. But he was not done yet. Brimming with confidence, he stepped out of the dugout, grabbed his bat, and took a few practice swings in the famed Fenway on-deck circle before entering the batter's box. He stared down at home plate, the same spot where Red Sox catcher Carlton Fisk had homered in the 1975 World Series, the same spot where David Ortiz had helped lift the dreaded Curse of the Bambino in 2004 in a comeback win against the New York Yankees before ultimately capturing the World Series title, Boston's first since 1918.

The history was not lost on Pete. He stared back at the pitcher, a player he had been having his way with all day. The Harvard hurler wound up and released the ball over the plate. It was exactly where Pete wanted it. He swung at the pitch with all the strength he could muster. The loud crack of the bat echoed through the small crowd. The ball sailed over the pitcher's head and kept going. Pete watched as it continued to rise before eventually landing in the Fenway bullpen. John, Nancy, and Andrew were on their feet with hands raised triumphantly in the air. They hugged tightly with the realization in the back of their minds of the long journey that had taken Pete from his boyhood home in Beverly to Boston College. Pete smiled broadly and pumped his fist as he rounded the bases and was met at home plate by his overjoyed teammates. The Eagles beat Harvard 10–2 to capture the coveted Beanpot trophy, which Pete lifted high over his head in the middle of the sacred outfield. He was named Most Valuable Player of the tournament.

That night Pete and his teammates went out celebrating around the Chestnut Hill campus. There was no shortage of drinking holes near Boston College, but one place was off-limits to all athletes: the infamous dive Mary Ann's. The dingy Cleveland Circle bar sold dollar draughts and was notorious for underage drinking, fights, and blackout binging. It had such a bad reputation that Boston College coaches uncompromisingly barred their players from going there.

But Pete and his teammates had celebrating to do, and Mary Ann's was a Boston College institution, after all. They had a fantastic night, hoisting the Beanpot trophy in the air, drinking from it, doing shots and taking pictures with it. Pete and his pals got away with the rule violation, and five years later—after Hughes was long gone and coaching at Virginia—Pete sent him pictures of the Beanpot behind the bar at Mary Ann's. Hughes had a good laugh.

For Ryne Reynoso, one of his most cherished memories during that junior season came in the locker room, not on the field. One Saturday Ryne went down to Alumni Stadium, where the team's small locker room was located, and was planning to get his gear to go work out at the batting cages. When he entered the locker room, he was stunned. Pete stood in the middle of the locker room wearing nothing but his batting gloves and cleats, with a whiffle-ball bat, hitting balls off of a tee.

"What the hell are you doing?" Ryne asked.

"Naked dry hacks, man. Naked dry hacks," is all Pete said, as he went back to smacking whiffle balls around the locker room.

Coach Hughes's success in the ACC did not go unnoticed nationally. Virginia Tech was able to lure him away in the summer of 2006. Pete was heading into his senior year, and the coach who recruited him—his mentor and friend—was leaving. It was hard for Pete to accept, but Hughes's replacement was Mikio Aoki, a BC assistant coach from Plymouth, Massachusetts, who had played college ball at Davidson College with Hughes.

"It's an awesome feeling to be the head coach at Boston College," Aoki said upon his introduction. "This program has had a great deal of success under Coach Hughes. . . . BC is definitely a program on the rise."

Aoki named Pete captain and spoke highly of him, telling reporters, "Pete brings a ton of energy to our team. He's a leader and plays incredibly hard. He's improved immensely during the past couple of years. He's an outstanding athlete who has made himself into a very good baseball player."

Pete also graced the cover of the team's 2007 media guide.

In addition to losing Hughes, Ryne Reynoso also left Boston College after he was drafted by the Atlanta Braves as a pitcher. Ryne struggled with the decision to skip his senior season but ultimately chose to go to spring training in Orlando, Florida, after BC's 2006 season ended. He never made the big leagues but played a few years of Triple A ball in the Braves farm system, including a year in Portland, Maine, where Pete was a regular visitor.

Pete's senior season rivaled his junior year, as he again led the team in home runs, with five. He also stole twenty-two bases and set a Boston College record with eight RBIs in one game. He went 4-for-6 in an April 14, 2007, game at the University of Maryland, including a grand slam, a three-run home run, and an RBI double. It was a strong ending to his college playing career, and Pete was feeling optimistic about his prospects of continuing to competitively play the game he loved.

8

THE DIAGNOSIS

Upon graduation from Boston College in 2007, Pete took an entry-level job as an analyst for EMC, a large technology and data company. He had just started work when an old BC baseball buddy called about an opportunity to extend his playing career overseas. He was hungry to play but felt he could not turn his back on his new job. Instead, he recommended his best friend, Tommy Haugh, who had just wrapped up his playing career at Bentley College. Tommy played that year in Europe and had such a life-changing experience that he begged Pete to join him the following season.

Pete had been toiling away in a thankless job on the lowest rung of the corporate ladder, but his thoughts were never far from baseball. In fact, he thought that he would audition for a minor-league team and asked one of his college coaches to assess his skill set for the pros. Mike Gambino had been an assistant coach at BC and was now serving in that same role at Virginia Tech under Coach Hughes. Gambino ran Pete through a series of drills before he eventually determined that Pete did not have the right stuff for professional baseball in the United States.

"You don't have enough power in your bat or strength in your arm," Gambino said, matter of factly.

Pete appreciated the honesty, although it pained him to hear it. He had made giant leaps as a player from high school to college but had hit the ceiling before reaching the next level. Still, he wanted to play ball and Europe was calling.

He soon joined his friend Tommy in Germany, where they lived together and played together for the Hamburg Stealers. A few months before Pete's departure, John had purchased tapes from Rosetta Stone to help his son learn the language. Pete refused to listen to the tapes. John found the stubbornness curious, as his son had always prided himself on his preparation.

"I was even more surprised when I visited him in Hamburg a few months later," John remembers. "Pete had learned all the German phrases in a brief period of time—especially the swear words."

In short time Pete had also taken control over the team. He was a player-coach, and he ran the team's youth program to teach German kids how to play America's national pastime. Pete had immersed himself in the local culture and made friends easily among both the American and European players. He was by far the best player on the team, but, as he had done at Boston College and St. John's Prep, he made it his mission to elevate and nurture his teammates. The German coach praised his German players for their discipline, but with discipline came a habit for overanalysis. If a German player hit a double, he would run to first base and stop to assess the situation before heading to second base. Pete taught the German players to feel the game naturally and play with a little more reckless abandon.

When Pete returned home a year later, he brought with him a snobbish taste for German beer and a German knack for opening bottles with anything but a bottle opener, including a rolled-up newspaper. He teased his dad for drinking god-awful Bud Light, but after being home a few weeks he rediscovered his appreciation for domestic brew.

Needing to find work quickly, he took a job selling group insurance. It was time to join the real world, but Pete knew early on that he was not cut out for a typical nine-to-five corporate job. He had voiced his frustrations to Nancy during that family getaway to Florida. He was now in an emotional and professional slump, but, just as he had done in baseball, Pete knew that he would have to play himself out of it. He grew even closer to his dad at this time.

"Both of us worked in Boston, talked every day, and had lunch at least once a week," John recalls. "He'd come home on weekends, and we'd tackle projects around the house together, watch sports, and just talk. When he'd leave on Sunday, I'd always stand outside no matter the weather and wave furiously as he drove away. I just wanted to make sure he felt the love."

Pete's other lifeline during this time was his budding romance with Julie, whom he had met during a preholiday pleasure cruise on July 3, 2011. That afternoon Pete, an old friend from St. John's Prep named Henry Pynchon, and a group of buddies headed to a sprawling waterfront home in Marblehead to hang out with one of Henry's college pals, who had a yacht tied up along the shore. The boys planned for a daylong excursion to Brown's Island off the coast of Gloucester, a popular party spot for twenty-somethings from the area.

The boat was loaded with beer and food, and the guys had music blaring as they pulled up to Brown's Island and tied up next to some friends. Before long there were twenty-five boats tied together, creating one giant floating party. Young men and women climbed from boat to boat, mixing and mingling, dancing, doing shots, and soaking in the sun. There was no shortage of gorgeous young women, but one group stood out, especially to Pete and Henry.

There was a group of four girls, all wearing stars-and-stripes bikinis. One of them was Julie Kowalik, a striking Boston College senior from Marblehead. Out of all the girls on the boats that day, Julie, with her silky blond hair, athletic build, bright smile, and dark tan, was the one driving all the guys crazy. They all took their swings with Julie and her friends but struck out. The women were not interested.

"I'm gonna go talk to her," Pete said.

"Dude, no way. No chance," Henry said.

"Watch."

Pete was chiseled and handsome, but his buddies liked to tease him that he had "no game" with the ladies. He was normally very nervous and shy around girls. The guys were sure Pete would be coming back dejected in no time, but Pete was brimming with confidence on this day.

He managed to infiltrate their circle and got right to Julie. They hit it off, much to the amazement of his pals.

"What the hell?" Henry observed. "How is he even talking to her?"

"You're Andrew Frates's brother, right?" Julie asked Pete.

He smiled. All through their lives, Andrew had always been known as Pete's brother. But Andrew had become quite popular in college, and now the roles were reversed. They chatted and Pete got her phone number. He realized immediately that he had met someone special.

Pete and Henry were both working in downtown Boston at the time and met for lunches regularly. Henry often called Pete at his desk and was always struck by the fact that Pete changed his voice mail daily. While most people had a generic "I'm not in, please leave a message" greeting, Pete updated his daily, specifying the day and a specific greeting based on his day-to-day schedule.

Sometimes Pete would pick him up in his black Mercury Milan—which Pete nicknamed "The Lucic" after former Boston Bruins star Milan Lucic—blaring Iron Maiden with the windows down and sunroof open. Pete would be bellowing out the lyrics as he pulled up, drawing glares from the buttoned-down business lunch crowd, which only encouraged Pete more.

A few days after the boat bash, they met to grab a sandwich and discussed the holiday party.

"Dude, that girl was so hot," Henry said.

"That girl from Marblehead? I'm going on a date with her," Pete said.

"Yeah? That girl in the stars-and-stripes bikini?" Henry asked.

"Yep," Pete said proudly, biting into his sandwich.

"Good for you."

As attractive as Julie was, she did not have many boyfriends. She stayed single for the most part while at Boston College, preferring to maximize her fun and friendship with her girlfriends rather than get bogged down in a relationship.

Julie's parents, Joe and Kate Kowalik, first heard about Pete shortly after he and Julie met. Kate's niece had gone to BC with Pete's sister, Jenn. So when a family friend called Kate and said, "I heard Julie is seeing Jenn's little brother, Pete. That's so cute," Kate was a bit shocked.

"Cute my ass," she told her husband. "He's twenty-six years old. She's only twenty-one."

Kate was also concerned because Pete was a popular, handsome athlete and she was protective of her daughter. In her words, she was concerned Julie would just be "the pretty girl of the week." But then they met Pete and heard Julie talk about him. It was clear from the beginning that there was a deep connection and a true love blossoming.

The Kowaliks were first introduced to Pete at a college football game in the fall of 2011. Pete wore his customary tailgating outfit, which included a maroon vest and a tie.

"Dear lord, what is this kid wearing?" Kate said to her husband.

But Pete acted like a true gentleman and quickly showed his sense of humor and straight-forwardness.

"So, when you were on that boat, Pete, how did you pick which girl with the American flag bikini to ask out?" Joe asked him.

"It was easy," Pete said. "I chose the one that was over twenty-one, and I could buy a drink for."

Joe, who played baseball at Cornell University, took an immediate liking to Pete, as they talked about the Red Sox, BC, and Pete's city league team, the Blue Sox.

The Kowaliks knew their daughter was fearless, but they also knew she had a temper when she got mad. It did not take long before Kate and Joe felt protective of Pete, as though he was their own son, and took to playfully reminding Julie, "You be nice to him!"

The bond between Pete and Julie grew quickly. While Pete was immersed in his job and was assimilating into postgraduate life in South Boston, Julie allowed him to keep a foot in the college world and Boston College, where she was working on her degree. Julie spent much of her senior year at Pete's place in South Boston, but there were many weekends spent in Chestnut Hill, where she was able to enjoy her senior year, and Pete was able to let loose on campus and relive his glory days.

At one tailgate during Boston College's pathetic 2011 campaign, Pete, Henry Pynchon, and Julie and her friends had a tailgate so epic that none made it into the game, which was not all that unusual during a season that saw the team go 4–8 under Coach Frank Spaziani. The guys and girls got separated, and Pete and Henry wandered "the mods"—a college housing complex of four-bedroom duplexes in the heart of the campus—drinking, carousing, and reveling in a carefree afternoon. Nature called as they meandered aimlessly, so they headed back to Julie's room, where they found the girls and decided to host an impromptu redecorating party. The guys found some pink spray paint, and soon Pete's name was emblazoned across the walls. The girls joined in, drawing faces and scrawling their names. It was harmless fun and a favorite memory for Pete and Julie, even though she and her roommates wound up having to repaint the whole room.

Still, despite her natural beauty, Julie was awestruck that the Boston College sports hero had taken such an interest in her. But after hanging out with Pete and listening to him butcher a heavy metal song during a night of karaoke, Julie quickly realized that Mr. All-American had a goofy and playful side to match her own. The two became inseparable, and each began to dream about building a perfect life with the other. Things were moving along perfectly.

But then that night at the Blue Sox game, Pete was hit by that pitch. *That pitch.*

He had not felt the same since. The pain in his wrist lingered and would not go away. Soon, the discomfort began to spread. "I started to feel a twitch in my upper arms," he recalls. "I thought, okay, I'll drink an extra Gatorade, eat an extra banana, and be okay."

He attempted the remedy, one that always allowed him to bounce back quickly from a sports injury in the past. But this time, it did not work. His illness had begun to manifest itself in different ways. He suffered from mood swings brought on by stress and fatigue. Pete tried to keep up with the rigors of his job. He was on the road constantly meeting with clients across New England.

"I'd get on the road at six in the morning and plow through six meetings during the day," Pete recalls. "All my life I had energy to spare, but now I was growing tired very fast." His sales job often took him to Hartford, Connecticut, about a hundred-mile drive from his apartment in South Boston. Halfway there Pete would get consumed by fatigue. He would look for the nearest rest stop, pull in, and sleep.

"I felt so bad, literally sleeping on the job," he says. "But my body was so exhausted. I worried that if I didn't pull over, I would crash." Pete did not let anyone else know what was happening to him because he had no answers for himself. "This was my secret and I didn't want to let on that the soreness in my wrist was just the tip of the iceberg."

Julie started seeing signs that had her concerned about Pete. For one, he was sleeping late all the time. When they first met, he would get up by five o'clock to go work out, but these days he was struggling to get up by eleven. He was also having trouble buttoning his shirts, and when she stayed over in his South Boston apartment, she often found herself helping him do the simplest of tasks. He always loved to cook for Julie, but that started to be too much for him. One night he spent all day picking up meat, fish, and vegetables and was exhausted by the time he got back to the apartment. He asked her to help him cook, because he just could not physically do it.

Another evening, during a walk home from a neighborhood bar in Southie, Pete suddenly became legless and needed the assistance of his buddies to make it back to his apartment. The next day his friends joked about it.

"Dude, you were pretty bent last night," one of his friends laughed.

Pete did not see the joke.

"I wasn't drunk last night," he confided to them. "Something's wrong. Something's happening to me."

Pete retreated to his bedroom alone and opened his laptop. He could not explain to his buddies, to Julie, or even to his parents how he was feeling. The Internet search browser came up, and Pete took a deep breath. His fingers trembled. He began typing his symptoms into the computer—muscle spasms, fatigue, problems with coordination, weakness.

He hit ENTER and waited. Pete's heart pounded as the Google search engine went to work gathering and collating the appropriate links. The first to appear was a link to the ALS (amyotrophic lateral sclerosis) Association website. The ALS Association defined the disease as a "progressive neurodegenerative disease that affects nerve cells in the brain and the spinal cord." The term *amyotrophic* was an amalgamation of Greek words. "A" means no. "Myo" means muscle, and "Trophic," refers to nourishment.

No Muscle Nourishment.

The disease attacked the nerve cells responsible for controlling voluntary muscles in his arms, legs, and face. The website described particular symptoms that included difficulty walking and struggling to button one's shirt.

"It was if they had put a camera on me over the last few weeks because that's exactly what I was experiencing at the time," Pete recalled.

The website also offered a list of notable individuals who have been diagnosed with ALS. The first name Pete read was Lou Gehrig. Because he was a fellow baseball player, Pete instantly recognized the name. Gehrig, a legendary first baseman for the New York Yankees and baseball Hall of Famer, died from the disease, as Pete recalled.

Pete's forehead began to sweat, and his mouth went dry. But he read on to discover that ALS was a rapidly progressive disease with no cure. ALS was invariably fatal.

FATAL.

Pete closed the browser window and retyped his symptoms once again. This had to be a mistake. The search engine spat out another list of websites.

Each listing began with three simple yet shocking letters—A-L-S.

He had worked his entire life to build a healthy body, and now his body was rebelling against him in the worst possible way.

The pitch that struck his left wrist had turned into the ultimate gut punch. Once again he gasped for breath, and tears began to form at the corners of his eyes.

How could this be? ALS *is an old person's disease. . . .*

As Pete wrestled with the uncertainly of his future in his mind, he thought about his life with Julie. "I kept thinking to myself, what will she say if I have to tell her that I have *ALS*? What will she do?" Pete remembers.

He also thought about his parents. Pete knew they would support him as they had done his whole life, but would the one-time college sports star become both an emotional and financial burden on his family?

He kept his pain and anxiety to himself, not wanting to hurt those he loved. Each ALS website had stressed that anyone diagnosed with the disease should get a second opinion. Quietly, Pete began scheduling appointments with doctors around the city of Boston. He told his family and Julie that he was simply getting his nagging wrist injury checked out. Nancy and John believed that it was nothing more than an orthopedic injury that could be corrected by routine surgery or possibly therapy. They were concerned that the wrist injury could affect Pete's ability to play the sport he loved, but that was it. The Frates family went about their daily lives, and that is exactly how Pete wanted it. Still, the emotional pressure was building inside of him, as doctors offered no clear answer as to what was wrong. They ruled out several possibilities, including Lyme disease, but they had not ruled out the one condition that Pete had feared most—ALS.

First, doctors began testing the nerves on his left arm—the infected arm, to shock the nerves and gauge his muscle fiber. They continued to poke and prod elsewhere, a needle behind his ear, another under his chin. They asked him detailed questions about his ability to walk and whether he had difficulty buttoning his shirt.

"I had a freak-out moment right there," he remembers. "Like me, the doctors were beginning to fear that I had Lou Gehrig's disease."

Several months passed and Pete's concern grew, as the disease continued to destroy his muscles slowly and methodically.

He finally shared his fear with Julie while the two lay in bed during a ski trip to Maine—a trip Pete knew would be his last. "I'm scared baby," he told her as she snuggled in his arms. "For the first time in my life, I'm truly scared about what's gonna happen to me."

Julie wrapped her arms around his stomach, squeezing him tighter.

"Whatever it is, we will tackle it together," she replied with a soft kiss to his shoulder. "I love you."

The words comforted Pete, but, inside, his mind raced, as he remained immersed in fear and doubt. Pete did not mention the dreaded acronym ALS to Julie that night. He would not speak of it until there was a formal diagnosis. Pete pulled Julie close and stared at the ceiling, waiting for sleep to come.

The Frates family received a visit from Jenn and her husband, Dan Mayo, a short time after. The couple traveled from New York City to share exciting news. Jenn was pregnant. John and Nancy were overjoyed at the idea of becoming grandparents for the first time, but Pete responded differently.

"I told my brother that he was going to have a little niece or nephew, but I didn't expect his reaction," she recalls. "He seemed sad. It was only later that I truly realized why." Jenn noticed subtle hints in Pete's behavior and his dexterity and realized there might be something more to his nagging wrist injury. "He was having a hard time cutting into a strawberry on the kitchen island. He couldn't hold the knife quite right."

The Frates household was filled with laughter and love that weekend, but Pete was sitting on a time bomb. Doctors wanted to see him. They had discovered what was wrong.

Pete had braced himself for the news but understood that it would blindside his family. He called his mother. "Mom, I have a doctor that has found a diagnosis for my nagging wrist," he told her. "Do you and Dad want to come to the appointment with me?"

"Of course," Nancy replied.

They arrived at the neurologist's office at Boston's Beth Israel Hospital a few hours later. Nancy and John had taken separate cars, as both were going to head off to work afterward. Nancy arrived late due to wet weather that had locked up traffic across the city. She entered the examination room, where Pete and John were waiting with two doctors. Minutes later two more physicians filed into the small room. Dr. Seward Rutcove, the chief neurologist, grabbed a chair, pulled it close to the family, and sat down.

"Well, Pete, we've been looking at all the tests, and I have to tell you, it's not a sprained wrist," Dr. Rutcove said in a sober tone. "It's not a broken wrist, it's not nerve damage in the wrist, it's not an infection, and it's not Lyme disease."

Nancy looked at the doctor curiously. *Where's he going with this?* she thought.

Dr. Rutcove placed his hands on both knees and leaned forward, staring directly into Pete Frates's eyes.

"I don't know how to tell a twenty-seven-year-old this. Pete, you have ALS."

Pete nodded in agreement, hearing the words he had hoped to never hear. The diagnosis was now official. However, Nancy and John did not fully understand. Nancy thought back to her own cancer diagnosis decades before. Surely, like other diseases, early detection of ALS meant a positive prognosis. Her husband was also hopeful.

"ALS? Okay, what's the treatment?" John asked.

"Yeah, let's go," Nancy added. "What do we do? Let's go."

Dr. Rutcove sighed as he turned his attention to Pete's parents.

"Mr. and Mrs. Frates, I'm sorry to tell you this, but there's no treatment, and there is no cure."

No treatment. No cure.

Nancy got up and ran out of the room. As she entered the hallway, her knees buckled and she collapsed onto the nearest chair, sobbing. "Oh my God, my son's going to die," she screamed.

Nurses surrounded her. John rushed to comfort her. Nancy felt like her heart had just been ripped from her chest. In her mind Pete was still the baby who had fought so hard to live after a staph infection. He was the naturally gifted adult with the physique of a champion. How could this be true? How could a disease like ALS affect her son? Nothing made sense. Nancy fought to regain her composure. The last thing Pete needed to deal with right now was a hysterical parent. She took several deep breaths and wiped away the remaining tears. It was time to be strong.

After several minutes she returned to the examination room and put on a brave face for her firstborn son. Still, the realization of Pete's fate was too much for Nancy and John to comprehend. They knew that both of them would not be going to work that day, and their future had suddenly shifted under a cloud of uncertainty. They drove back to the family home in Beverly and immediately called Jenn and Andrew to come home.

Andrew awoke that morning feeling tense. He knew his big brother had a big doctor's appointment and was not sure what was looming ahead. He was hoping for the best but feared his brother had a serious health problem. He never considered that Pete's problem could be terminal, but he was concerned that it could be something major that would change their lives.

"Good luck today," Andrew texted to Pete.

"Tx bro. Ttyl," Pete replied.

Later that morning Andrew was toiling away at his IT sales job when his phone vibrated and a text message came up from his dad: "you need to come home right now."

He stepped away from his desk and called John.

"What's going on, Dad? Just tell me what's happening," Andrew said.

"You need to come home. We're having a family meeting," John said sternly.

"Dad, what's happened to Pete?" Tears welled up in his eyes as he paced in the hallway of the sterile office.

"Just come home, Andrew."

The phone went silent. Andrew felt like he was going to pass out. His heart and mind raced. He was on the verge of a breakdown. He scurried into his boss's office and burst in, tears pouring down his face.

"I have to go, man. I'm sorry. There's something with my brother. He had a doctor's appointment, and they won't tell me what's wrong, but it's serious. My parents are never ambiguous like that. I just have to go. I'm sorry," he said.

He grabbed his work bag, sprinted out the office door to his car, got in, and hit the ignition. He raced from his office in Framingham toward the Massachusetts Turnpike and sped onto Interstate 95 toward Beverly with no regard for the speed limit and barely holding himself together on the forty-minute ride.

"What does Pete have? What are we dealing with? It's gotta be some form of cancer," he mumbled to himself.

When he arrived home, John and Nancy met him on the front porch. Both looked weary and had clearly been crying. Nancy gave him a big hug and squeezed him tight. She rested her head on his shoulder and whispered to him, "Pete has ALS."

"What? What's that?"

"It's bad, Andrew. Very bad," John said, holding back tears.

"Pete is resting upstairs, but he wants to talk to you," Nancy said.

Andrew waited for his brother. Pete came down after a few minutes and found Andrew in the kitchen, pacing.

Pete opened the sliding door and asked Andrew to join him on the back deck. It was a beautiful March day that was unseasonably warm. It was almost seventy degrees, and there was not a cloud in the sky. The two brothers sat in lounge chairs side by side, as they had done thousands of times to talk about sports, girls, school, friends, and their futures.

Pete explained to his younger brother that there was no cure and no treatment. He laid out, in stark terms, the harsh realities of ALS.

"It's going to attack my muscles," Pete told him. "You're not going to see this big strong guy anymore."

Andrew began to sob.

"Suck it up man. This ain't gonna stop us," Pete said. Andrew had seen that look in Pete's eyes before. It was one of determination and confidence.

It was the look he saw when Pete went to play a big game for Boston College or St. John's Prep. Andrew saw no fear in his brother's eyes. Only the steely-eyed gaze of a man ready for battle. Andrew fed off Pete's strength.

"We're gonna beat this thing," Andrew said, tears again coming to his eyes.

"We're getting to work, man," Pete said. "I'm putting my work boots on."

With that, he got up, hugged his brother, and headed to grab his car keys. He had to drive to Boston College to pick up Julie and tell her the news.

Pete sat in his car as it idled in the parking lot in front of Julie's dormitory. In his mind's eye, he could still see the look of fear and hopelessness on his mother's face from just hours before. Pete was sweating. He was about to tell the love of his life that he was stricken with a disease that could shorten his life span to just five more years. He had been given a death sentence, and he could not imagine sharing that burden with her. But he could also not imagine living the rest of his life without her by his side.

The front door of the dorm opened, and Julie stepped out, wrapped in a light coat, her long blond hair blowing in the March wind. She looked into the car and caught Pete's eye. Julie froze. She sensed something was wrong. Pete stepped out of the vehicle and called her over.

"Get in the car, baby. We need to talk," Pete pleaded.

Julie did not move.

"C'mon. Please get in the car."

She walked toward him. "Tell me. Tell me what the doctors said."

"I'll explain when we get back to Beverly," he replied.

Julie stood her ground. "I'm not getting in your car until you tell me."

Pete paused, trying to find the right words. "I'm sick."

"I know you're sick," she said. "How sick?"

He looked down at his feet, unwilling to meet her gaze. "I have ALS. I have Lou Gehrig's disease."

Taking a deep breath, Julie took a moment to process the news. "Take me home," she told him. Pete looked back up at her. He feared that she would have this kind of reaction, but he had resigned himself to the thought of losing her forever.

"You want me to take you back to Marblehead? I guess I understand."

"You don't get it," she replied. "I need to tell my mom that I'm leaving BC." Julie wrapped her arms around his neck. "And then I'm coming home to you. You are my home."

It was not what Pete had expected to hear. He thought she would ask for a little time to process the sobering news instead of committing herself to him instantly and with purpose. However, this determination had been recognized by Harvard scientists when she was just a toddler.

Julie was fearless.

_____

Jenn was back in New York City and stuck in an important meeting at work. Nancy did not want to interrupt her daughter and feared a dire phone call could potentially jeopardize her pregnancy. She called Jenn's husband, Dan, instead and relayed the news. Dan began Googling ALS for a quick tutorial of what the family was now facing and printed out some materials. He then jumped in a cab and headed for Jenn's work. He pulled out his cell phone and called his wife.

"I'm on my way to pick you up," he said.

"What do you mean?"

"I can't tell you right now," he said. "Just walk out to the street. I'm in a cab and I will pick you up."

Jenn got into the cab and her husband broke the news. "Pete has ALS."

She was confused. Jenn thought her husband was talking about a friend of theirs, not her brother.

Once she realized the truth, she began howling and screaming in the back of the taxi. "I can't believe this," she sobbed. "Not Pete. I just can't believe this."

They returned to their apartment in Brooklyn and packed their bags and headed for the airport.

During the flight to Boston, Jenn was catatonic. She could not move or speak. She thought back to the previous weekend at home with Pete.

She was surprised that he had agreed to an early morning breakfast with her instead of sleeping in as he normally would have.

"He knew what was ahead, but he wanted one more moment of normalcy with me," she recalls. "He knew that bad news was coming and I didn't. I think about that a lot and how difficult it must have been for him, and how happy I am that he did it. "

The Frates family gathered around the dinner table of their Beverly home. The clan was in a fog. Nancy passed a few dishes around, and John, Jenn, Dan, and Andrew took small portions to spread around their plates. No one spoke. Pete sat in a chair at the end of the table, watching. It was as if there had been a death in the family, and the departed had been invited to join them for dinner.

Pete Frates the captain, Pete Frates the leader, had to step up to the plate. "There will be no wallowing, people," he announced. "We are not looking back. We're moving forward."

Pete's voice was forceful. He spoke with authority. His parents and siblings all sat up straight in their chairs. A bolt of lightning had just illuminated the room.

"What an amazing opportunity we now have to change the world," Pete continued. "I'm going to change the face of this unacceptable situation of ALS. We're going to move the needle and raise money to fight." Pete explained that he was going to get out in front of this disease like no one had done before. "I'm gonna convince philanthropists like Bill Gates to get involved."

He had been a young man searching for a purpose, for a mission in life. He had now found it—or it had found him.

That night Pete made grand promises and commitments that could have seemed far-fetched for some, but Nancy and John knew their son was capable of great things when he put his mind to it.

A few short miles away, Julie was engaged in a different conversation with her own family. She had made a decision to leave college and an opportunity for a normal life to stand by and care for the man she had grown to love. "There's no me without him, and there's no him without me," Julie told her mother. "I love him. This is our life now."

Kate Kowalik heard strength and resolve in her daughter's voice, and it would have been impossible to talk Julie out of this life-altering decision.

Julie's mom gave both her blessing and support, helped her daughter pack her bags, and then drove her to her new home with Pete and his family in Beverly. Pete welcomed Julie with open arms, but he had one condition. He knew how hard she had worked, and he wanted her to finish out her senior year at Boston College.

"When we received the diagnosis, nothing else mattered to me than to be by his side, but Pete was able to see the bigger picture more clearly than I was," Julie says.

He would drive her daily to campus, where Julie's professors showed their support, giving her extra help and the tools she needed to graduate on time. While her classmates worried about entering the tight job market and perhaps finding a place to live upon graduation, Julie set her own goals.

On the night of the diagnosis, lying in Pete's childhood bed, surrounded by trophies from his past, the couple held each other close and discussed their uncertain future. Pete's mind raced about his newfound mission, while Julie had a mission of her own.

"I want to have a baby," Julie told him.

"With me?" Pete asked, only partly kidding.

"Yes with you," she laughed.

The conversation then turned serious. He placed his hands on her soft, delicate face. "Are you sure you want to be with me?" he asked. "You have your whole life ahead of you. You can do anything you want."

"Shut up," Julie replied. "I am going to marry you and have your baby."

Their's was an uncertain future, but there was no uncertainty in her words. They were not individuals any longer. They were one.

"And I thought that I was the determined one," Pete said happily.

9
MOBILIZING AN ARMY

The next morning Nancy awoke in a pensive mood. As she lay in bed, the morning light cracking through the skylight blinds, she thought back to her son's athletic career and how she and her husband made the conscious decision to attend every game Pete played. They never missed a single one.

"We weren't overbearing, like some other parents, though," John says. "We made sure that we had a positive or constructive comment after each game just to show him that we were paying complete attention and appreciated all the work he was putting in to get better."

They were there when Pete crushed a home run into the bullpen at Fenway Park. They were there when Pete was hit in the wrist by that fateful pitch—his last at bat.

There was a forty-five-year-old man on Pete's team, and Nancy always noticed that his parents were there at every game. "That will be me and Dad," she joked to Pete. "Sitting there watching you play when you're fifty years old."

It always made Pete smile.

These memories made Nancy smile too. She climbed out of bed and hugged her husband. "You know what, John? I'm not sure I can handle this at all. But I have no regrets."

Outside his immediate family, the first person that Pete notified about his condition was his best friend, Tommy Haugh. Tommy was down in Atlanta at the time working for a baseball facility. It was early in the morning, and Tommy was the only one there. His cell phone flashed with a FaceTime request from Pete. Tommy accepted and Pete appeared on the phone screen. He was sitting on the bed in his bedroom with Julie seated beside him. Both looked exhausted.

"What's going on here? Why aren't you at work, buddy?" Tommy asked with a nervous smile.

"Tommy, I've been going to the doctors a bunch, and I've been having some tests done," Pete said.

He paused. Tommy stared into his iPhone screen, looking into Pete's eyes.

"They've figured out what's going on. It's some sort of muscular disorder called amyotrophic lateral sclerosis. It's Lou Gehrig's disease."

Tommy was stunned. The only words he could manage were "I love you."

Pete continued to speak, but Tommy heard nothing but ringing in his ears. He was in shock. Both said good-bye, and Tommy hung up the phone to collect his thoughts. He took a deep breath and called his best friend back.

"Everything is going to be okay," Pete reassured him. "We're gonna figure this thing out."

Over the next several days Pete and Tommy reached out to former teammates and friends to quietly spread the word. Pete did not want those closest to him to learn about it secondhand or read about it online or in the newspaper. Mostly, he wanted his dearest friends to hear the strength in his voice.

Pete reached out personally to a former roommate named Mike Budreau. Mike had been aware that Pete had been undergoing medical tests for some time. Mike also saw firsthand how his pal was struggling to accomplish the simplest of tasks. One evening, just a few weeks before the diagnosis, Pete visited Mike's apartment, where the two friends had a few beers while playing a game with dice. Pete tried rolling the dice, but it kept falling out of his hands and onto the floor.

"I know your left hand is still screwed up from getting hit by the pitch," Mike said jokingly. "But your right hand should be fine, so quit screwing around."

Pete furrowed his brow and looked seriously at his friend. "I got something going on Boudy."

The smile disappeared from Mike's face. Later, just as Pete would do, Mike googled the symptoms, and he kept coming across articles about ALS. He prayed that that it was something else—anything else.

The night after Pete received official word, he called Mike, who was sitting on his couch with his girlfriend. Mike saw the number flash on his cell phone and answered immediately. Pete was matter-of-fact on the phone. His voice was confident and reassuring.

"Hey Boudy, I wanted to give you a call to let you know that I have ALS," Pete said. "If you google it, you'll find some not-so-great stuff."

Pete did not know that Mike had done research on his own and knew what his close friend was facing.

"I could barely speak," Mike recalls. "My throat had a baseball-sized lump in it, and my goal was not to let Pete hear me cry."

Pete continued, "We're making some calls now and letting people know that we're gonna start fighting this thing." He spoke with conviction and his words provided hope to his good friend.

"His positive attitude was unmatched," Mike remembers. "I believed right then that if anyone had a shot of beating this unbeatable disease, it was Pete."

Pete also called Coach Hughes, the man who had taken a chance on him at Boston College years before. Hughes was coaching Virginia Tech at the time but remained a mentor and close friend to Pete. Hughes had gotten a heads-up from a Boston sportswriter that Pete was sick but did not want to jump to any conclusions until he talked to his former player directly. That happened as Hughes was on a bus trip en route to play Georgia Tech, when he got a call from Pete.

Pete broke the news but immediately tried to put his coach at ease.

"Don't worry. Coach, I've known I've had this thing for over a month," Pete told him. "I went into the doctor's meeting and knew what they were going to tell me. I just wanted to be there for my parents." He continued, "I want to be the face of this disease. There's a reason why I'm so young and got diagnosed with it. Because I can get out there and speak. I want to get out there and captivate people and get some momentum for this disease. I'm going to change this disease forever."

Hughes listened, a lump in his throat, thinking about the difficult road ahead for a player who had become one of his favorites. The bus rumbled down Interstate 85, Hughes's current players blissfully clueless as to the heart-wrenching conversation unfolding on their coach's cell phone. The coach paused, chose his words carefully, and told Pete, "If there's anyone more equipped to beat something they give you no chance to beat, it's you. Because of your toughness and your attitude."

Carly Nardella was a neighbor in Beverly who had dated Pete when they were just kids. When she heard the news, she texted her childhood crush immediately and told Pete that she loved him. Like many, Carly struggled emotionally with the realization that her strong, kind friend was very sick. "Everything I was reading about ALS was the complete opposite of how I envisioned Pete," she recalls. "As a young male, he was an outlier, and I thought, coupled with his athleticism and active lifestyle, he was somehow going to beat this mysterious disease."

When Carly heard back from Pete, he sounded like he was very much in control of the situation. But when she met with Pete, Julie, and some other friends for drinks later that week, Carly noticed that he was having trouble putting money back into his wallet. As time went on, she saw more glaring examples of his physical breakdown and knew that she had to do something to help.

Later that week Pete and Julie met some friends for dinner in Marblehead. It was a couple's night right around Saint Patrick's Day, so they decided to head out for an enjoyable evening like they had so many times before. The friends, Jay Connolly and his girlfriend, Nicole Benson, noticed that Julie did not touch a thing on her plate during dinner. After the bill was paid, they moved to the bar downstairs and found a table near the fireplace. Against the warm glow of the burning logs, Pete filled them in about his uncertain future.

"Guys, listen to me for a sec," Pete said. "I wanted to get you together here so I could tell you something that is going on with me. As you know, I've been having trouble with my wrists. After many doctors' visits, it turns out that I have this thing called ALS."

Nicole started to cry. She was a nurse and understood how dire the prognosis was. Julie broke down in tears also and both left the table to console each other outside.

Jay was fighting back tears of his own but he stayed at the table with Pete.

"Jaybird, I don't want you to get upset," Pete told him. "We're gonna strap up the boots and keep going. This is what we're going to do!"

Jay put on a brave face for Pete, as Nicole did later. But when they returned home from dinner that night, the couple wept in each other's arms for both Pete and for Julie.

Pete continued to confide in a small circle of friends, lifting each one of them up, urging them not to feel sorry for him and telling them that he would enjoy his mobility for as long as he had it. Soon that circle grew, as more friends mobilized for Pete and reached out to his vast network of former Boston College teammates.

Ryne Reynoso was fighting for a roster spot at spring training for the Cincinnati Reds in Phoenix, Arizona, when Pete called him. But Pete had forgotten that it was his friend's birthday and did not want to ruin his day.

"Have fun with the family and call me in a few days to catch up," Pete said.

Two days later a mutual friend and fellow teammate informed Ryne of the situation.

"I leaned back in my locker pulling some shirts over my face to hide the sadness," Reynoso recalls. He had always thought the worst day of his life would be the day that he could no longer play professional baseball. Reynoso was cut by the team that spring. He says the anguish over losing his job and his dream was nothing compared to the real possibility of losing his baseball brother and close friend.

Joseph Ayers, the utility player from Alaska whom Pete had taken under his wing after he transferred from Stanford, echoed the disbelief of those who saw Pete up close in the gym and on the ball field. "How is this possible?" he asked himself upon hearing the news. "He's a monster, one of the strongest guys in the weight room on our team." Ayers sought spiritual guidance because the reality of the situation made little sense to him. "Every time I'm in church, God and I have a little conversation about what's going on up there. I hope one day I get to find out why stuff like this happens."

Pete's physical strength was a direct byproduct of thousands of hours spent running, throwing, and lifting weights. But he now had to rely on a greater power, his inner strength, to see him through. He was handed a virtual death sentence, but he refused to let it kill his adventurous spirit.

Pete did not allow the disease to get in the way of his immediate plans, which included attending a bachelor party with friends in Austin, Texas. He was not going to slow down. A buddy asked what he would like to do while visiting Texas. Pete wanted three things—to go to an Iron Maiden concert, to catch a Houston Astros game, and to take a ride on a boat. He wasn't into pleasure cruising. Pete wanted to go fast.

They met up at a lake, and Pete's pal had gotten them a ride on a cigarette boat. Pete's eyes lit up when he saw the sleek vessel, one built for speed. They jumped in the boat and the driver pushed the throttle. Moments later the boat was topping speeds at ninety miles per hour. Pete requested a life jacket because he could not grip the rails as tightly as he used to. His pal strapped him into the life vest and interlocked his arms with his own. Soon they were off again and having the time of their lives.

All of Pete's close friends experienced a mourning phase filled with bouts of sadness, anger, and disbelief. Their only comfort came from the one man who refused to give up or give in. Pete began to form a battalion made up of friends and loved ones who would take his lead and join the mission to wipe out ALS. To fight back, Pete's army had to learn more about amyotrophic lateral sclerosis and more about the legendary ball-player whose name has come to symbolize the deadly disease.

10

NEW YORK, 1939

The day was April 30, and over two hundred thousand spectators had gathered at Flushing Meadow Park to get a glimpse of the future. It was a particularly hot Sunday for midspring, but the soaring temperatures did not dampen the collective spirit of those attending the grand opening of the New York World's Fair. The exposition had promised visitors a look at the world of tomorrow.

A new technical marvel called television was introduced to the masses by RCA with its special broadcast of President Franklin Delano Roosevelt's opening speech. Albert Einstein piqued great curiosity among learned attendees with his talk about cosmic rays. But the biggest draw was an exhibit sponsored by General Motors called Futurama. The attraction provided a redesign of the American landscape, as visitors were shown what the country would look like in twenty years time, when an inter-connecting highway would transport people and commerce from one side of the United States to the other by automobile. General Motors supported the idea for the simple fact that more roads would allow the company to sell more cars to consumers. This innovation would also mark a rapid decline for America's most popular mode of transportation at the time—the locomotive, the iron horse.

Twelve miles away a much smaller crowd of just over twenty-three thousand had gathered at Yankee Stadium in the Bronx. They were not there to see the future. Unknowingly, they were there to witness the end of an era.

It was a routine play, one he had made countless times over 2,130 consecutive games in the major leagues. But Lou Gehrig's once-powerful legs had trouble gathering momentum. A Washington Senators player bounced a ball toward pitcher Johnny Murphy, who had to hold onto it for a few precious moments while Gehrig lumbered over the first base bag to field the throw. The putout play was successful, but just barely. Disgusted by his own play, the Yankees legend took himself out of the lineup for the next game against the Detroit Tigers on May 2, thus putting an end to the longest streak for consecutive games played in the history of major league baseball. The record would stand for fifty-six more years, but Lou Gehrig's days were numbered.

His mind was clear, but his body was breaking down rapidly. Lou Gehrig was no longer the man who could crush the ball, hitting forty-seven home runs in a single season or four homers in one game. He was no longer the player who could steal home like he had done a whopping fifteen times during his career. His physical strength was legendary, and his stamina and durability were almost superhuman. Gehrig's endurance had earned him the nickname, "The Iron Horse."

He was born strong. He was the only child born to German immigrant parents who had survived infancy. Henry Louis Gehrig was born in 1903 in Yorkville on the Upper East Side of Manhattan, which at that time was a working-class neighborhood crowded with immigrants from Ireland, Poland, Hungary, and Germany. His mother, Christina Fack, worked as a laundress and cooked and cleaned for others. His father, Heinrich, was a steady drunk who landed the occasional job as a metal worker.

Their son took to sports early and was a natural athlete with particular prowess on the football field and baseball diamond. After starring in both sports at New York's Commerce High School, he was lured to Columbia University to carry the pigskin as a member of the school's fearsome backfield. He chose to play baseball there instead. He joined the Phi Delta Theta fraternity but felt ostracized because of his working-class background. His mother sometimes cooked for the fraternity brothers to earn extra money. By extension, Gehrig was treated like "the help" and would never be welcomed into the fraternity's well-heeled social circles. Young Lou found his true home on the ball field, where every man could become a king with enough dedication and skill.

In April 1923, on the very day that Yankee Stadium opened its doors,

Gehrig pitched a game for the Columbia Lions against Williams and struck out seventeen batters. A Yankees scout was in the stands that day and worked to sign the collegiate phenomenon to a big-league contract less than two months later.

Lou Gehrig made his professional debut in June 1923, when he was just nineteen years old. He earned a spot on the team as a pinch hitter before cracking the starting lineup at first base in 1925. A year later he scorched the league with forty-seven doubles, twenty triples, and more than one hundred runs batted in. He also hit sixteen homers, earning the respect of his teammate Babe Ruth.

From there he was as dependable as daylight. He played every game with a tenacity and fury as if it were his last. The statistics were staggering, and the accolades came pouring in. Gehrig won the Triple Crown in 1934 and was named league MVP in 1927 and 1936. He was selected to the All-Star Team for seven consecutive years and helped lead the Yankees to six world titles. *Time* magazine proclaimed him the game's "no. 1 batsman" and one who "takes boyish pride in banging a baseball as far, and running around the bases as quickly, as possible."

Lou Gehrig was maniacal about his sport. "I am a slave to baseball and only because I love the game, hate to think of taking even one day off when we are playing," he said. He also had a high tolerance for pain. No matter what injury he had endured on the baseball field, rest was never an option. There was the time when he was struck in the head by a pitch and nearly rendered unconscious but stayed in the game. There was the time that he was hit by a pitch just above his right eye and knocked out cold, yet was in the lineup the very next day—and this was just exhibition season. He had suffered numerous concussions both on and off the field, including a postgame fight with Ty Cobb, where he took a hard swing at the Detroit Tigers great, but missed. Gehrig fell and cracked his head on the pavement, knocking himself out. Several years later when doctors x-rayed his hands, they discovered that he had broken them in seventeen different places and kept playing while his hands healed.

Mortality began to creep its way in during the 1938 baseball season, when Gehrig found himself struggling at the plate and in the field. His batting average fell below .300 for the first time in a decade, and his slugging percentage was down. This would merely be considered an off year by normal baseball standards, but Gehrig recognized that his body was changing. He complained that he grew tired by midseason and just could not get going again. The problems followed him off the baseball diamond as well. His wife, Eleanor, noticed that Lou was having a difficult time tying his shoes. He now wore tennis shoes that he could slip easily on and off his feet. His physician thought Gehrig was suffering from a gallbladder problem, so they placed him on a diet of bland foods. He continued to grow weaker.

When the 1939 season came around, the Iron Horse had become a shell of his former self. He played only eight games and made just four hits. On May 2, 1939, the Yankees had traveled by train to Detroit to take on the Tigers at Briggs Stadium. It was customary for the team captain to deliver the lineup card to the umpires. Gehrig climbed out of the visitor's dugout and made his way toward the officials and handed them the card. The umpires scanned the lineup, and they were startled to see that Gehrig's name was missing. Ellsworth Tenney Dahlgren, also known as "Babe," was penciled in at Lou's spot at first base. The lineup card was then delivered to the public-address announcer, who understood the gravity of the moment.

"Ladies and gentlemen, Lou Gehrig's consecutive streak of 2,130 games played is over," the announcer told the stunned crowd of eleven thousand fans. The Yankees thumped the Tigers that day by a score of 22–2. "Babe" Dahlgren homered in the win.

The decision to take himself out of the lineup and away from the game he loved crushed Gehrig, who cried before the game. A day later he sent a handwritten letter to his wife, in which he described his despair: "My sweetheart . . . that thing yesterday I believe and hope was the turning point of my life for the future as far as taking life too seriously is concerned. It was inevitable, although I dreaded the day, and my thoughts were with you constantly—how the thing would affect you and I—that was the big question and the most important thing underlying everything. I broke before the game because I thought so much of you. Not because I didn't know you are the bravest kind of partner but because my inferiority grabbed me and made me wonder and ponder if I could possibly prove myself worthy of you. . . . Seems like our back is to the wall now, but there usually comes a way out. Where and what, I know not, but who can tell that it might not lead to greater things. Time will tell."

The couple had been married for about six years. Eleanor Twitchell came from a wealthy family in Chicago, and she had caught Gehrig's eye during a trip to Comiskey Park. The two began a long-distance courtship until they married in 1933. She attended all his home games and had watched him sacrifice his body for his teammates and for the fans of New York. Eleanor vowed to remain close to his side as he faced the next challenge.

The team sent Gehrig and Eleanor to the Mayo Clinic in Rochester, Minnesota, where he underwent a battery of tests. At first, doctors told him that he was suffering from chronic poliomyelitis, commonly known as polio. Gehrig was prescribed medication, but the drugs had no effect. Physicians at Mayo Clinic then corrected their diagnosis. They told the Yankee star that he was stricken with a rare disease called amyotrophic lateral sclerosis. They explained that his muscles were getting no nourishment from nerve cells in his spinal cord and that his body was wasting away. The chances for survival they said were about fifty-fifty.

These odds were outrageously high, and Gehrig's body continued to break down, as his muscles degenerated quickly. He was treated at Mount Sinai Hospital in New York and would have disappeared quietly from view had it not been for a popular sportswriter named Paul Gallico, who suggested to the team that it should plan a day in Lou Gehrig's honor. The Yankees chose July 4, 1939—Independence Day.

Gehrig did not want a day of recognition. He did not want to reveal that he had a disease or to show the public how thin and sick he looked and truly was. But he was a good Yankee and, as captain of the team, he allowed the event to take place. Fans thanked him by filling sixty-one thousand seats in Yankee Stadium to see him and possibly hear from him for one last time. Babe Ruth and other teammates from the 1927 Yankees squad that had won 110 games and a World Series championship were on hand for the ceremony. New York City mayor Fiorello La Guardia showed up to honor the Iron Horse, as did other dignitaries. But the fans themselves were only interested in seeing number 4—Lou Gehrig. After trophies and other honors were handed out to Gehrig, it came time for him to speak.

Something kept Gehrig from moving toward the row of microphones. There was a moment of awkward silence before the crowd was finally told that he would not be addressing them on this day. The microphones were about to be removed from the field when Yankees manager Joe McCarthy, a close friend of Gehrig's, whispered something into his ear. Gehrig then moved quietly forward, and, without the accompaniment of any notes, he addressed the crowd.

"Fans, for the past two weeks you have been reading about a bad break I got. Yet today I consider myself the luckiest man on the face of the earth. I have been in ballparks for seventeen years and have never received anything but kindness and encouragement from you fans. . . . When everybody down to the groundskeepers and those boys in white coats remember you with trophies—that's something. When you have a wonderful mother-in-law who takes sides with you in squabbles with her own daughter—that's something. When you have a father and a mother who work all their lives so you can have an education and build your body—it's a blessing. When you have a wife who has been a tower of strength and shown more courage than you dream existed—that's the finest I know. So I close by saying that I might have been given a bad break, but I've got an awful lot to live for."

Gehrig remained with the team for the rest of the season, watching from the dugout as the Yankees captured another pennant, this time against Cincinnati. Eleanor Gehrig then took her husband back to their home in Riverdale, where he worked for the parole board as a favor to Mayor La Guardia. But it was the mayor who had given Gehrig a gift—the gift of doing something noble for New York City. Eleanor would drive Lou to his appointments with prison inmates in an effort to determine whether they had rehabilitated their lives and were worthy of parole. Gehrig enjoyed the work, although he admitted to knowing virtually nothing about criminology. But his body continued to collapse on itself, and even the most menial tasks proved to be giant struggles. Eleanor did what she could to keep his spirits up—she never mentioned that he had a fatal disease. Instead, she entertained her husband with impromptu performances from Broadway stars in their living room. When he was alone, he listened to music and opera.

On June 2, 1941, less than two years after his diagnosis, Lou Gehrig died in his sleep, just shy of his thirty-eighth birthday.

Later, when asked about the burden of caring for her husband in his final years, wife Eleanor simply said, "I would not have traded two minutes of the joy and the grief with that man for two decades with another."

11
THE STATS GEEK

Seventy-two years had passed since Lou Gehrig made his inspirational farewell speech at Yankee Stadium, and scientists were still virtually no closer to discovering a cure for the disease that bore his name. Gehrig's legacy endured through film in the 1942 *The Pride of the Yankees*, starring screen legend Gary Cooper; several books; and numerous television documentaries. The average person had heard of Lou Gehrig's disease, but very few had any understanding of what it was and what it did. Therefore, research funding was painfully slow and could not keep up with the speed of ALS, as it aggressively ate away at the bodies of the afflicted.

Pete had studied the old film clips of Gehrig's speech and noticed little subtleties, such as the fact that when the Iron Horse was given several trophies and plaques, he never held them in his hands. Instead, he guided them to the ground, because his arms were not strong enough to hold them. Pete also saw that Gehrig's balance appeared to be fragile, as he moved very slowly and methodically during and after the ceremony.

"You could have put me in that film, and it would have looked the same, felt the same," Pete told a video crew from ESPN. "The disease is the exact same as it was all those years ago, so I think—what's wrong with this picture?"

On average fifteen people are diagnosed with the disease each day in the United States and about thirty thousand Americans may be currently living with ALS. That number is miniscule compared to the 1.6 million people that are diagnosed with cancer each year in the United States.

As insidious as amyotrophic lateral sclerosis is for patients and their families, the fact that it affects only a small percentage of the population makes funding for research an insurmountable challenge. It is a double-edged sword. On the positive side not many people are faced with the horrific disease, while on the negative side its rarity breeds a lack of attention. Certain events, such as the Persian Gulf War, caused brief spikes in research funding. In 2013 Congress allocated $7.5 million to fund the ALS Research Program at the Department of Defense after a surprisingly high number of veterans were diagnosed with the disease. That same year Washington spent $4.3 billion on cancer research.

Undaunted, Pete and his family decided they were going to get right down to the business of finding the best medical team in the world. Knowing that Boston was renowned for its hospitals, they felt confident they would connect with the brightest doctors and researchers who were on the front lines in the war against ALS. John and Nancy Frates began working their vast network of professional and personal connections.

John had many cousins who were among Boston's medical elite, but rather than turn right to them, he instead recalled an article written by *Boston Globe* sports columnist Dan Shaughnessy about his own daughter, who had cancer. In the column, Shaughnessy, an infamous curmudgeon and constant thorn in the side of players—especially the Red Sox—recalled how Sox legend Ted Williams read his column about his daughter and reached out to the sportswriter. Williams famously despised Shaughnessy, along with the rest of the media, but put that aside to help a man in his darkest hour. Shaughnessy forged a relationship with Williams, and the Splendid Splinter helped connect the writer to some of the best cancer doctors in the city.

John was now hoping that the *Globe* columnist would pay his good fortune forward. This would not be a cold call from a stranger. Pete had played baseball with Shaughnessy's son at Boston College, so they had a connection. John had his phone number and placed the call. He was a bit surprised when Shaughnessy picked right up. John told Shaughnessy the grim diagnosis and asked him for advice on what to do.

"I'll tell you what. I have this great relationship with Larry Ronan, the head doctor at the Red Sox," Shaughnessy said. "Let me call Larry and I'll get right back to you."

Moments later Shaughnessy called back and pointed John in the direction of Dr. Merit Cudkowicz, chief of neurology for Massachusetts General Hospital at Harvard University and one of the top ALS doctors in the world. But the family had one problem. They had been informed that Dr. Cudkowicz was not taking any new patients.

"The best ALS doctor in the world was in our own backyard, and we couldn't get access to her," John says. "But we were not going to be denied."

The Frates then mobilized Pete's friends to bombard the good doctor with phone calls and e-mails requesting an appointment. They were successful. On the day of Pete's first appointment, John, Nancy, Julie, Andrew, Jenn, and her husband, Dan, all crowded into Dr. Cudkowicz's office at Mass General. The doctor greeted the family with an air of cool professionalism. She had had been on the front lines of this horrific disease for several years and had learned not to give patients of their families false hope. She did kick off the meeting with a bit of humor, though. "Of course I will treat Pete. So can you please call off the dogs?"

The family laughed.

Dr. Cudkowicz explained that only about 10 percent of ALS cases were the result of some inherited genetic defect. The cause of the remaining 90 percent, known as sporadic ALS, was still a mystery. The ALS doctor then began to ask Pete a list of questions. "When did you take your last bowel movement?"

Pete answered. Ordinarily, family members leave the room when such personal questions are asked, but the Frates were not going anywhere. They wanted to understand everything.

Once again, Pete was taken from examining room to examining room and run through a battery of physical tests. One nurse sat on Pete's legs and attempted to pry them apart. "I've worked with everyone, professional athletes and the like," she told Pete. "I always break them."

He laughed. She pushed harder and he laughed more. She eventually gave up. She could not break Pete.

After several hours of grueling physical exams, Pete and his family returned to Dr. Cudkowicz's office. "How close are you to finding a cure?" he asked her.

"We still know very little about ALS," Dr. Cudkowicz replied, with just a hint of an Italian accent. "To find a cure, we need the proper funding for research. Right now, we are working with less than $3 million per year, compared to $25 million for AIDS research. Meanwhile, hundreds of thousands of patients around the world are losing their lives to this disease."

"How much do you need?" Pete asked.

"Look, Pete, it's my job to get donors, okay?"

He would not waver. "I'm not kidding around. How much do you need?"

The doctor quickly ran the numbers in her head. She placed her hand on his knee. Her tough exterior was beginning to melt. "I dunno, Pete. Probably a billion dollars."

Pete was unfazed. "I'm gonna get working on that," he told her.

———

Being a former baseball player, Pete was a typical stats geek. The statistics never lied. He soon learned that the average human being lived for approximately 28,502 days. He also learned that most ALS patients live for only 1,000 days after diagnosis. But Pete understood that stats do not tell the entire story. They cannot measure the heart of a person or their will.

"It's 2012, not 1939, when Lou Gehrig gave his final speech at Yankee Stadium," Pete would tell others. "There are a lot of people out there doing a lot of great things, and people who know me well enough know that I'm not gonna take this thing lying down."

Pete's heart was strong and his mind was sharp, but the disease was gaining control over his body. A month after the diagnosis, Nancy and John saw the first signs of just how fast ALS was attacking their son. Pete was carrying his laptop and a few other things down the stairs when he lost all strength in his legs, tumbled down, and spilled onto the floor in the foyer of the family home.

"I heard the crash and went running to Pete," Nancy recalls.

She saw her once-strong son lying as helpless as an infant on the cold tile floor. "I'm calling 911," she panicked.

Pete shook his head in frustration. "No, Mom. It's fine. I want Dad to come and pick me up off the floor."

"What? Come on, Pete. He's in Boston. You can't stay here until he gets home," Nancy responded. "What if you're hurt?"

"Mom, I'm fine. I just want Dad here to help me up."

Nancy called John, who dropped everything and sped back to Beverly. He rushed into the house and found his oldest son lying in the foyer, with a pillow under his head, courtesy of his mother, working away on his laptop. John picked up his son, hugged him, and made sure he was steady on his feet.

"Thanks, Dad," Pete smiled.

John lay awake in bed that night. He could not get the image of his son lying on the floor out of his mind. "It's not how it's supposed to be," John told Nancy. "I'm a fifty-four-year-old guy watching his gracefully gifted son wither away. That's not how this is supposed to work."

A few weeks later Pete was again walking down the stairs—this time carrying nothing. His legs gave out again, and he tumbled into the foyer once more. The disease was ravaging his calves. Pete and his parents realized that he was losing his balance and motor skills even faster than the doctors had predicted.

John called work that day and quit.

Pete's soul searching led him back to a place he's always held close to his heart: the ocean. He was creating his bucket list—things he wanted to do and enjoy until the day came when, like all ALS patients, he became a prisoner in his own body. He and his friend Jay Connolly had spent many summers fishing and boating off the coast of Marblehead. Jay's family had a sprawling waterfront estate along the town's rocky coast, and Pete and Jay had taken full advantage of the easy ocean access on many lazy postcollege weekends. He and Jay had many afternoon chats on the Atlantic about one day buying a boat. There was never a rush to achieve this goal, as the buddies expected a lifetime of endless summers, but that all changed when Pete was diagnosed. The future was now. They scoured the Internet for Seacrafts—a high-quality starter boat they decided would be perfect for them as a first vessel. It became a pet project and a welcome distraction from all of the doctor's appointments, medications, and associated ALS business.

Pete was showing more visible signs of the disease and his speech was slurred, but he was still able to walk well enough to get on and off boats.

They looked at one in Connecticut and another on Cape Cod, but the boats did not suit their needs.

In January 2013 they found the perfect pleasure craft in Cape May, New Jersey, a small seaside town south of New York, about a six-hour drive south from Boston. They decided to make a weekend of it and brought Julie and Jay's girlfriend, Nicole, whom he later married, along for the trip. They drove down Interstate 95, dropped the girls off in Manhattan for shopping, and continued on to Cape May. When they saw the boat, it was love at first sight.

They drove back to Manhattan and met the girls and had a night out on the town with several of their Boston College friends who were living in the city. The next day, on the ride back to Boston, Pete and Jay made a deal over the phone and bought the boat. They already had a name: the *Screaming Eagle*, a tip of the hat to their alma mater.

For the rest of that year, the boat was all Pete could talk about. They kept it in the Frates yard in Beverly, where Pete enlisted his dad to paint the hull.

"What am I, the boat boy?" John joked.

But John, of course, happily pitched in, while Jay and some friends waxed the boat. Pete supervised meticulously and paid close attention to detail. When the weather turned warmer, they planned a christening and brought the boat by trailer to Kernwood Marina, a public boat ramp in nearby Salem along the Danvers River. The Frates, Julie's parents, and Jay's parents, along with Nicole and Julie, all came down for the big launch. Standing on the dock, Julie cracked a bottle of champagne on the hull, and everyone had a glass of bubbly, as Pete, Andrew, and Jay hopped in and shoved off.

Pete could barely contain his excitement. It was chilly on the water, but Pete did not care. He was just happy to be in his element and on his very own boat for the first time in his life. As they pulled away from the docks, Pete was able to drive and had a huge smile stretched across his face. Later, when his mobility confined him to a wheelchair and then a power wheelchair, it became impossible to get him on the boat. But their friends and neighbors with bigger boats in Beverly and Marblehead pitched in, making time to bring Pete out onto the ocean. Watching Pete's condition deteriorate was agonizing for friends and family, yet his resilience and refusal to quit inspired them throughout his battle. Still, he needed a good deal of help, getting up out of chairs, walking from room to room, and even going to the bathroom. His condition had not yet gotten to the point where he needed full-time nurses or caregivers, so friends and family filled that role. One day Jay and Pete were hanging out at Jay's house when Jay went to help his pal off the couch. Jay lost his grip and Pete slipped, falling hard to the floor with a loud crash, just missing hitting his head on the coffee table.

"Shit, are you okay?" Jay asked, horrified.

"Take it easy, man. I'm all right," Pete assured him.

Pete was flat on his back and could not move to get himself up. Jay was panicked as he tried in vain to pick his friend up off the floor, but ALS was unforgiving. Pete was deadweight. Jay reached under Pete's arms and tried again and again to lift him up. Jay was frustrated. Pete quietly coached his friend. "Take it easy, one step at a time," he said calmly. "We'll get me back on the couch."

Both were exhausted when they finally reached the sofa. Jay felt defeated. He could barely help his friend in this time of need. But he had to remind himself, *I'm the lucky one*, Jay thought. He needed to remain strong for Pete. There was no room for negativity in Pete's world. When others voiced discouragement at the sad, sobering reality of his condition, Pete put his rally cap on and spoke optimistically about how he was going to overcome ALS.

"When I beat this thing, I'm going to show the world that science is no match for the human spirit," he said. "We are unlimited in what we can do if we have the drive to do it."

There was no quit in Pete.

Jay and Pete shared a special bond, not only because they had gone to college together and loved to fish and boat, but because their significant others, Julie and Nicole, had become best friends also. In 2012 the couples decided to travel to Paris together for a weeklong trip. The idea was to go while Pete was still able to travel comfortably. The trip also marked the first time Pete had to use a wheelchair.

Nancy and John drove the four to Boston's Logan Airport, pulling up to the curb in front of the international terminal to see them off. Pete was having serious trouble walking and made the call to use a wheelchair. It would be easier on Julie and their traveling companions.

It was hard enough for John and Nancy to see Pete off for the trip, given all that was happening, but seeing him leave in a wheelchair, Jay pushing him, brought tears to their eyes. "This was his future," Nancy recalls. "Seeing your once-healthy son in a wheelchair made us sad and angry."

In Paris the couples stayed at the W Hotel and traveled across the city, visiting the Eiffel Tower, Notre Dame, and other sights, while stopping at outdoor cafés to sip wine and watch people. Pete savored each glass of wine, each slice of cheese and bread. He created these sensory memories so that he would be able to draw from them when he was no longer able to eat or drink. His consumption of France's rich food and fine wines took a toll on his changing body. While at a bar across the street from their hotel, Pete and Jay had a couple of drinks, and then nature called.

"Dude, I have to pee," he told Jay.

The disease had made it impossible for him to control his bladder. Pete had to urinate, and he had to go now. The only problem was that the bathroom was located down a long flight of stairs. Pete would never make it in time. Jay helped him off his stool, and Pete was uneasy on his feet. The bartender looked over curiously, as he thought Pete was drunk.

"There's no way we're going down all those stairs," Jay said. "There are about thirty steps."

"Yeah, that's not happening," Pete agreed. "Dude, I gotta go now. We're going outside."

As Jay helped Pete out of the bar, patrons began to laugh. Like the bartender, they thought that the young American had succumbed to too much French wine. Once they stepped outside, Pete's bladder gave way, and he began to urinate in his jeans.

"Dude! Take my pants down now!" Pete yelled.

Jay propped Pete up against a utility pole and pulled down his friend's pants, and Pete stood there on a busy Paris street, relieving himself for all to see.

Pete's utter embarrassment was soon replaced by laughter, as the two friends began howling at the absurdity of the situation. They had become the *Ugly Americans*.

12

HEROES EMERGE

Pete poured himself into his new role as a passionate and inspirational proponent for ALS funding and research. It was a role he had been preparing for his entire life. Like a candidate on the political stump, Pete spent weeks and months reaching out to friends and strangers, asking them to join his campaign—a campaign to save lives. He was tireless in his pursuit of a cure, despite bouts with fatigue that stole his energy and a near-total collapse of his muscles that made it difficult to stand and virtually impossible to walk under his own strength. Still, he felt blessed. He met with his old friend and coach Mike Gambino, who had recently returned to Boston College to lead its baseball program.

"Mike, I really just think I have a great opportunity here," Pete told the coach. "I'm young; I'm in good shape. I'm way younger than the average person with ALS. I think I can have a platform here. I'm gonna be the one to get people talking about this and gets us moving toward a cure."

Pete sat down with local newspaper reporters and reached out successfully to national media outlets to educate them on the plight of ALS patients like him and the lack of funding for researchers committed to discovering a cure. During an appearance on the *Charlie Rose Show*, the host asked Pete how he looked at the future, knowing that his prognosis was dire.

"My outlook on the future is very unclear," he replied. "I had plans of grandeur of having a family, the white picket fence, things of that nature. Right now, that's not certain for me."

Pete's honesty and his efforts got the attention of advocacy groups across the nation. One group, the ALS Therapy Development Institute, which touts itself as the world's foremost drug discovery center focused solely on ALS, presented Pete with its major award in 2012. The award was named for Steve Heywood, an architect from Newton, Massachusetts, who was diagnosed with ALS in 1998, when he was just twenty nine years old. Heywood would become the subject of a popular book, titled *My Brother's Keeper: A Story of the Edge of Medicine*, written by Jonathan Weiner, a recipient of the Pulitzer Prize. Like Pete, Heywood used his affliction to raise awareness for the disease. Heywood lived with ALS for eight years. His death in 2006 was the result of an accident caused by a detached respirator. His brother James, a mechanical engineer at MIT, had founded the ALS Therapy Development Institute in his honor.

Steve Heywood had carried the torch for his fellow patients and their families for nearly a decade. That torch has now been passed to Pete. He accepted the Heywood Award during a gala at the Sheraton Hotel in Boston. Dressed in a maroon Boston College polo shirt, he walked slowly to the podium, with the help of his dad and Julie, to enthusiastic applause.

"I always am so impressed and marvel at the people who go to work every day with the sole occupation to find treatments to make lives like mine a little better every day," he said with slurred speech. Pete called the researchers "heroes" for selflessly battling an unforgiving and formidable opponent like ALS. He then publicly thanked his family for the first time, especially Julie, for their loving support and their commitment to the cause and to him.

"It's coming down to a matter of dollars and cents," Pete told the crowd. "If we can get enough money into ALS research, I don't see why we can't make ALS go the way of polio and other diseases that we so fortunately have gotten rid of. I'm confident and hopeful that we can make ALS a thing of the past, and at one of these events we can just have a big party to celebrate the ending and the curing of ALS."

Like he had done in locker rooms in both high school and college, Pete created hope with his words. There were smiles in the audience and a sense of pride and accomplishment among the attendees.

His acceptance speech was followed by a panel discussion among biochemists, clinicians, and pharmaceutical executives. Nancy and John sat in the audience, following the conversation with rapt attention. As the discussion wore on, Nancy found herself lost in a labyrinth of scientific terminology.

"I tried listening, but most of the content shot way over my head," she recalls. "I avoided every science class in high school and college, but I knew body language, and I could tell that these panelists were unfamiliar with one another."

The researchers appeared to be working in silos, where compartmentalization stymied progress.

Nancy quickly raised her hand. "I'm Pete Frates's mom. First, thank you very much for working on ALS; it means so very much to us. But I'm listening to what you're all saying, and there doesn't seem to be a lot of collaboration going on here. Not only that, but where's the flip chart with the action items and the follow-up and the accountability? What are you going to do once you leave this room?"

The room grew silent. The attendees turned their attention to the panel members. The collection of experts had nothing to say.

Later in the hotel lobby, Nancy voiced her grave concerns to her husband. "Did you see that, John? She asked, dumbfounded. "They have no plan. They are treating this like an academic exercise, while our son is dying. It's almost like they feel that it's a hopeless cause."

Nancy and John saw it as a sign that they needed to drastically raise the level of fund-raising. More money would mean more resources, and more resources would help bring about a greater chance for a scientific break-through. The family had begun to organize small fund-raising events, but the donations, while welcome, were a drop in the bucket. The big question remained. How could they raise money on a mass scale to fight ALS?

Meanwhile, Pete was soon placed on an experimental "compassionate use drug," an investigative drug that was outside of a clinical trial. To receive it, Pete's doctors had to contact the pharmaceutical company, while also submitting an application to the FDA. They also had to agree that their patient, Pete Frates, had no other options. The drug was in a phase 3 trial. It was hope in a bottle for the ALS community, but it did nothing to slow the progression of the fast-moving disease.

Pete would have to search for his own remedies. He spent countless hours reading articles, white papers, medical journals, and other materials for information about ALS. It was all-consuming. One place his research led him to was medicinal marijuana. Pete had smoked weed in the past, but it was not high on his list of vices. He enjoyed his Budweisers much more than a joint, but he also was not judgmental and was fine with people enjoying a bong hit or two.

He learned that medicinal marijuana could have some benefits to ALS patients. Studies have shown marijuana can prolong the survival of brain neurons, and the plant's active ingredient, THC, has antioxidative, anti-inflammatory, and other neuroprotective effects that can help ALS patients. Pete knew the science was debatable, but he also knew he had nothing to lose and needed something, anything, to help him cope with the rapid, painful changes to his body. He had been suffering severe anxiety and muscle spasms, which he hoped the pot could help alleviate.

He rang up a friend and asked him if he could bake a batch of edibles for Pete to try. The friend was happy to oblige and baked a dozen brownies for him to eat. Pete did not want to try it alone. There was only one person he trusted enough to sample them with him—his brother, Andrew.

Andrew had also quit his job to be a full-time caregiver for his big brother. He had put his own future on hold for the brother he had idolized growing up. Pete's dreams now became Andrew's dreams. They both wanted Pete to get better, and both strived to find funds for a cure for ALS. Pete and Julie now lived in an accessible, in-law apartment that was built as an addition onto the Frates' Beverly home. All the materials used to build the two-bedroom addition were donated by area businesses, as was much of the labor.

One morning they woke up, and Julie had left for the day. Nancy and John also were not home, so Andrew and Pete had the entire house to themselves.

Holding the bag of brownies up, Pete said to his brother, "Dude, you want to do these?"

"If you're doing it, I'm definitely doing it," Andrew replied.

There was a sense of mischievousness about the whole thing. Their parents were not home, and they were about to do something that was against the rules.

They each ate a whole brownie but felt nothing after fifteen minutes.

Twenty minutes, twenty-five minutes went by and still nothing. They considered eating another, but then, suddenly, the brownies kicked in.

The brothers started giggling at nothing. They felt warm and happy. Pete was relaxed and felt fantastic, the woes of his body's deterioration faded away.

Pete made his way to the stereo and turned on one of his favorites: Iron Maiden. Andrew did not love heavy metal like his brother, but the vibe of the moment was infectious. Pete banged his head along with the thrashing sounds of Nicko McBrain, Steve Harris, Dave Murray, and Adrian Smith. He wailed along, singing every word along with vocalist Bruce Dickinson, hoisting his hands to the sky in time to the triumphant lyrics.

"Run, live to fly, fly to live, do or die," Pete shouted along. "Won't you run, live to fly, fly to live, Aces high!"

Andrew had tears in his eyes, and his stomach knotted from laughing so hard as they thrashed around the living room. Soon Julie arrived back home.

"Dude, Julie's home. Chill," Pete said. Like misbehaving little boys, they assumed seats on the couch, trying to hold back the giggles.

But that didn't last long. They began chuckling at each other.

Julie watched the commotion with a raised eyebrow. "What the hell is wrong with you two?" she asked. "You guys are up to no good." She looked over toward the counter and noticed the bag of brownies. "Oh my god, you guys are stoned off your asses!" she said, joining them in laughter.

They both giggled in agreement and Pete went back to the stereo and turned Iron Maiden back on. Julie's tastes were much more subdued, but, like Andrew, she too embraced Pete's heavier side and thrashed along with them.

———

Pete found freedom and motivation in music. He formed a relationship with members of Pearl Jam, his favorite band, thanks to his friend and fellow ALS warrior, former New Orleans Saints player Steve Gleason. The defensive standout made his name on the field for blocking a punt against the Atlanta Falcons during the Saints' first game in the New Orleans Superdome after Hurricane Katrina in 2006. Five years later in 2011,

Gleason was diagnosed with ALS, at thirty-four years old. Gleason had a young wife and a baby on the way. When Pete was diagnosed with the same disease the following year, he reached out to Gleason for advice and friendship. The two athletes hit it off immediately, and Gleason invited Pete down to New Orleans to participate in an ALS summit in 2013. While there with Julie and Andrew, Gleason brought them backstage to see Pearl Jam perform at the Voodoo Festival.

Pete was overjoyed as he sat backstage, behind the drum kit with Gleason, watching the band play to a massive crowd. Pete, Julie, and Andrew sang along, hugged, and laughed. With Gleason by his side in a power wheelchair, Pete screamed the lyrics to "Alive" and sang along pensively to the ominous "Black." Singer Eddie Vedder introduced Gleason and Pete to the crowd, eliciting wild applause. Lead guitarist Mike McCready at one point walked over to them and played the outro of "Yellow Ledbetter," hugging them both as he ended the song.

Gleason was struck by Pete's spirit and commitment to fighting ALS and bringing it out of the shadows. "Pete is an incredible guy, and I am so proud of him," Gleason told the *Seattle Times* after the concert.

It was a memorable trip for Pete, Julie, and Andrew. Pete's condition was worsening, but he still had some mobility and could talk, laugh, and, most important, sing. They hit Bourbon Street with a group of friends, and Pete enjoyed the atmosphere. At one point, as they continued down the busy thoroughfare, a group of guys at a bachelor party called out to Julie, waving her to come join them at the patio bar. Being a beautiful, young blond, it was not uncommon for Julie to draw male attention, so she knew how to handle it. She was in full party mode, though, so she made her way over to the group and joined them for a shot. Pete watched with a smile on his face, as Julie captivated the group with her beauty and charm. She enjoyed her drink and then rejoined Pete to continue their strut down Bourbon Street, kissing him softly on the cheek. Pete was proud of his wife, and it was yet another reminder of just how much he loved her. She was attractive, she was fun, and she was his. "That's my girl," he said, kissing her.

13
TOGETHER FOR LIFE

Pete's legs grew weaker by the day, and walking just a few short steps became as grueling as running the Boston Marathon. He now spent most of his time confined to a wheelchair. For Pete, it was not only humbling but maddening. The Frates were regulars at the Sterling Center YMCA in Beverly, which was run by Nancy's sister, Judith Cronin. Pete and John took a swim class that included water therapy for Pete. John wheeled his son in for the class. In the elevator John ran into an old friend whose daughter had recently beaten cancer. There was an awkward silence in the elevator, as the two dads locked eyes, each feeling the other's pain of having a sick child.

"How's it going?" the friend asked John.

"We're doing the best we can," John replied.

Pete interrupted, curtly and boldly proclaiming, "We're doing great."

As they left the elevator, Pete was agitated. "Dad, I don't want to hear you say anything like that again. We're always great," he said. "Always."

"Got it, Pete," John said.

It broke John's heart to see his son in a wheelchair, his health deteriorating before his eyes. John and Andrew had taken over many of Pete's life skills. Eating and drinking became increasingly difficult for him. He choked on his food often, and a simple meal turned into a difficult chore lasting up to an hour even with the help of his father and brother. But that was not the worst of it.

"Feeding, bathing, toileting, and dressing Pete for the first time were traumatic events for me," John says. "I kept remembering him as this big, strong 225-pound guy who was now down to around 200 pounds of deadweight. He felt tremendous pain if you moved him the wrong way."

The family had to count the number of calories Pete ingested every day. If he could not take in the required 2,500 calories on a given day, Nancy would make him a milkshake packed with protein powder and a packet of instant breakfast.

When John told the father of another young ALS patient that he quit his job to care for his son, the other dad was shocked. "Why would you do that?" the man asked.

"Pure love," was John's only reply.

Pete's message was clear from the beginning to John and everyone else that there was to be no one feeling sorry for themselves. And putting on a brave face, despite the dire circumstances, were the marching orders from Pete from then on.

Still, there were times when the family had to be honest with themselves and others about what they were dealing with. During a visit, one of Pete's old colleagues sidled up to John in the kitchen and asked quietly, "So, John, how's it going?"

Unaware that Pete was standing nearby, listening, John expressed his feelings.

"It's unbelievable to me. It's unfathomable this guy is suffering in a way that's so cruel," John started. "He did everything he could athletically. He took care of his body. It was the cruelest of all the diseases, because now it's his body letting him down. It's a tragedy."

Pete was incensed and got in John's face right there in the kitchen.

"Tragedy is a word reserved for children dying prematurely and soldiers coming home in body bags," Pete scolded. "Don't ever use that term again to describe my situation. I don't want to hear that word used again in this house."

Later, after all the friends had left, John and Pete had a talk, and John apologized for offending him.

"So what word is acceptable, Pete?" John asked.

"I don't know. Devastating, horrific, terrible," Pete said. "Those are okay. But never tragedy."

Once again Pete refused to dwell on his own condition. But when he did voice concerns, he spoke only about how his disease affected his loved ones, especially Julie.

"I know it's not easy," Pete confided to his closest friends. "I'm sure she never thought she'd be taking care of her twenty-eight-year-old boyfriend who walks around like he's ninety."

Although he was now stuck in a wheelchair, Pete was determined to use his legs for two of the most important moments of his life—walking Julie back down the aisle after becoming husband and wife and waltzing with her for the first time as a married couple. But first, he would have to find the perfect ring to propose with. He called his sister, Jenn, and confided in her. She offered him the ring that had belonged to their great-grandmother, which was in her possession. It was a cherished family heirloom, and it was now a symbol of the family's love for Julie.

John and Nancy still had no idea what was happening. A few days before the engagement, Pete was inducted into the Inner City League Hall of Fame in Boston. Once again he used the platform to talk about ALS. Toward the end of his speech, Pete stated that he would be the first Hall of Fame inductee to come back and play in the league. The crowd was lifted to its feet as they showered him with applause. It should have been a great evening, but Pete was feeling agitated. John asked him what was wrong, but Pete said he did not want to talk about it.

In bed that night, he wrestled with his decision. There was no doubt that Julie was the love of his life and that he wanted to marry her. She had been unwavering in her love and commitment to him, but a ring would cement their relationship for life, however long that lasted. It was the last chance for him to let go and let the woman he loved walk away and enjoy a more comfortable, more complete life. He hated to rob her of those moments that every couple should have the opportunity to experience.

His own daily routine was growing progressively worse. He began soiling their bed, as muscles could not hold in his waste. He appeared drunk when he walked, and his speech was now a collection of slurs. His body was getting ravaged by the disease. *Is this what she truly wants?* he thought to himself. *I was once Superman. Now I need to be monitored and cared for like an infant.*

Oblivious to Pete's inner turmoil, Julie, half awake, rolled over and hugged him tightly. With a sleepy smile, she whispered, "I'm so in love with you."

She fell back asleep and Pete's heart soared. They were not individuals any more; they were indeed one.

A couple of nights later, at the Frates house, Pete asked Julie's father, Joe, to step outside with him, telling him he wanted to show him his new boat. But there was another reason he wanted to talk to Joe alone.

"You know how much Julie means to me," Pete said to Joe. "I love her so much, and I'd like to marry her."

"You're asking me for my daughter's hand in marriage, and I give you approval for that," Joe said.

With Joe Kowalik's blessing, Pete popped the question a few nights later. Earlier in the evening, John helped his son get ready for dinner.

Pete's hands were not working.

"Dad, can you go over to my drawer?" Pete asked. "Push the socks aside, and you will find a ring box. Can you put the box in my pocket and get Julie and ask her to come in?"

John did as he was asked and fetched Julie. She entered the bedroom and closed the door. Pete's dad gathered Nancy and told her what was happening. Moments later there was a sound of hysterical crying coming from the bedroom, followed by joyous laughter.

John and Nancy were thrilled with the idea of welcoming Julie into their family. Julie's parents shared in that excitement, although many family friends came forward to voice their misgivings.

"They would say, how can you let your daughter do this? She's only twenty-one years old. She's got her whole life ahead of her," Joe recalls. "They were understandable questions, but these people didn't understand Julie or the love that she and Pete had. It was unconditional in the strictest sense of the word."

Julie's mother agreed. "There wasn't a moment I thought I could talk her out of this, even if I wanted to," Kate remembers. "It's Julie. If I had said anything to her other than 'I'm completely here for you,' she would have said to me, 'Don't talk to me again until you tell me what I need to hear.'"

The Kowaliks kept their fear for their daughter's welfare to themselves. Joe had struggled with Pete's diagnosis from day one. He wished the doctors all got it wrong and that maybe Pete just had a severe case of Lyme disease or perhaps multiple sclerosis. At least then there would be some hope for the future.

But as acceptance turned to reality, Joe took a different approach. He would define hope in a different way. He had hope that Pete could live a full life, despite the disease. He had hope for a cure and hope for better treatment. If hope one day fell short of reality, Julie's parents would have had time to live life with Pete, share in their happy times, and truly live in the moment.

Joe told his daughter as much. His father had fought in World War II, so Joe knew firsthand of the sacrifices made by soldiers. Many of them were Pete's age, or frequently younger, when they went off to war, never to return.

"There are many hard things for kids to deal with at age twenty-two," he told Julie. "ALS is a tough one, but you're surrounded by people who love you. We need love and we need hope. For many people in my father's generation, young guys went off to war and never had that hope. There's still some ingredients here for us to still have hope."

Pete also tried to brace his future wife for the long road ahead. "It's gonna get worse before it gets better," he told Julie.

She said she was up for the challenge, but in her heart she struggled. Julie put on a brave face for Pete, but privately she asked herself, *Haven't we had the worst yet? Can it get better now? It's so hard watching the man you love so much. His body is failing, and there's nothing I can do about it.*

Pete comforted her. "My body may be failing, but my mind has never been more focused," he said. "I see things more clearly now. I observe things, like the blue sky, trees, in a way I never saw them before. I see our bond, our love, which only grows stronger each day."

—

The wedding was planned for June 1, 2013, and preparations got quickly underway. Julie brought her mom and Nancy shopping and drove from boutique to boutique for the perfect dress. Nothing truly caught her eye, until they stopped at a small bridal shop in Beverly. They did not have an appointment. They walked in and told the owner they were merely browsing.

"I had no intention of buying my dress there," Julie remembers. "I tried on one dress and then another. Once I tried on that second dress, I knew that it was special." She turned the corner from the fitting room and swept into the parlor with the white dress cascading to the floor. The mere sight brought Nancy to tears. Julie was the most stunning bride she had ever seen.

Pete would be in for a pleasant surprise when he saw her on their wedding day. Meanwhile, the groom-to-be was working on his own big surprise. He reached out to the athletics staff at Boston College to see if it was possible to have the BC marching band play at the wedding. It would be a BC affair, after all, since the bride and groom both bled maroon and gold, as did most of the wedding guests. The staff members loved the idea and secretly coordinated with Pete over several more weeks.

Julie had no clue.

The family finally had something happy and positive to celebrate. They had all been living under a dark cloud of despair and uncertainly since the diagnosis. But as they planned for the wedding, Pete and his family never took their eyes off the ball.

In February 2013 Pete and Nancy traveled to Silver Springs, Maryland, to speak before the U.S. Food and Drug Administration. The FDA panel included a who's who of the federal government's top decision makers when it came to experimental drugs to treat ALS and other rare diseases. It was the FDA's first-ever public hearing on amyotrophic lateral sclerosis. The topic at hand was the agency's regulations on drugs for the treatment of ALS. Despite his physical condition, Pete was determined to travel to Maryland because he wanted the decision makers to see him in person—to see the result of the government's unwillingness to approve more experimental drugs and to bolster federal funding.

When it was time for him to speak, Pete demanded action and reminded the FDA panelists that patients like him could not afford to let time slip away.

"We all know the two-to-five-year life expectancy of a person with ALS," he said. "It's completely, utterly unacceptable. I ask of you, let's speed up the process. Let's work together and let's get this disease a thing of the past."

Pete received a round of polite applause following his testimony. Government officials said all the right things, but the Frates family soon realized that the FDA was a giant bureaucracy where the earth shifted slowly, if at all. How could they translate Pete's passion-filled words into action? The hourglass measuring the days, minutes, and seconds of Pete's life was tipped over, and time was running out.

—

Still, the wedding proved to be a welcome respite from the Frates family's mounting frustration. The morning of the ceremony, Julie and her brides-maids, which included Jenn, her cousins, and childhood friends, went to get their hair done at a salon in town. Julie was not experiencing any of the wedding-day nerves and jitters common with most brides. She was fearless, after all. The ceremony was scheduled for early evening, and she was counting down the hours with great excitement. While at the salon, she received a text from Pete.

"I know that I'm breaking the rules, and we're not supposed to talk," he wrote. "I just want to tell you how excited I am to marry you and see you at the church."

The emotion of the moment caught up with Julie, and tears began to form. She wiped them delicately away from her face as to not smudge her makeup.

The couple did not take any pictures together before the ceremony, as has become a custom for newlyweds in the new millennium. Instead, they wanted to keep it traditional. They wanted that magical moment in the church where they saw each other for the first time.

Pete had chosen his brother, Andrew, and Tommy Haugh to serve as his best men. Tommy wheeled Pete into the church, as the idea that he could walk Julie back down the aisle now seemed like a distant dream. In the weeks leading up to the wedding, he had lost nearly all the strength in his legs and had to be assisted when he tried standing up for short intervals.

Andy and Tommy each held onto Pete's elbows as he stood at the altar, dressed in a charcoal tuxedo and pink bow tie. Julie entered the church on the arm of her father. When Pete saw his bride, his eyes lit up and his jaw literally dropped.

Two Catholic priests performed the ceremony: Father Bill Schmidt, a family friend, and Father Anthony Pena of Boston College. Julie had not received Catholic confirmation, which would allow her to get married in a Catholic church, so Father Pena worked with her to make it happen in time for the nuptials.

When Pete and Julie stood to recite their vows, Pete's jacket was hanging awkwardly. He couldn't move his arms to fix it, so his pal Henry Pynchon got up from his seat and adjusted it for his friend. Nancy, sitting across the aisle, looked at Henry and mouthed, "Thank you."

The couple chose traditional Catholic vows. Pete and Julie pledged to hold each other from that day forward, for better, for worse, for richer, for poorer.

"I thought leading up to our wedding that I would become emotional when having to recite 'in sickness and in health,'" Julie remembers. "But when I was up there sharing this day with friends, family, and, most of all, Pete, I didn't flinch." *Fearless.*

There was no fear in her new husband either. They kissed deeply as the priests pronounced them husband and wife. The nearly three hundred guests clapped and hooted. Tommy positioned himself next to the wheelchair. Pete frowned at his co–best man. Julie spoke. "Are you ready?" she asked.

"I'm ready," he replied.

"What do you want to do?"

"I want to walk."

They turned to their guests with their hands clasped together. Andrew took Pete's other arm.

They proceeded down the aisle just like Pete had dreamed.

The wedding guests rose to their feet. The applause began slowly and, soon after, rose to a deafening roar. Pete stopped midway down the aisle and kissed his bride with the strength and passion of ten thousand men. They continued out of the church and into the sunset of early evening as Mr. and Mrs. Frates.

After the ceremony, the wedding party took a trolley to a nearby yacht club, where they boarded a lobster-fishing boat and cruised Marblehead Harbor, where Pete and Julie had first met.

The wedding reception was held under a tent at a waterfront estate in Marblehead owned by Jay Connolly's parents. The servers and bartenders donated their time for free. The band played for the bare minimum. Friends took care of flowers and place settings. The tables were named accordingly—Birdball, Shea Field, and so on.

The walk to the tent was a long one, but Pete managed with the help of Andrew and his bride. They entered the tent to the sounds of Hall & Oates, which was soon replaced by the ring of trumpets from the BC marching band playing the national anthem. Julie looked at Pete in amazement.

"How'd you pull that off?"

He smiled and shrugged.

"There's nothing like being in your favorite place in the world, having just married the man of your dreams with every family and friend that matters most to you," Julie recalls. "My cheeks actually hurt from smiling and laughing so hard. Pete and I made our way to the dance floor, where we were greeted by our bridal party in a big group hug."

Pete and Julie shared their first dance as husband and wife to the song "Somebody like You" by Keith Urban. "I've always been a big country fan, and we both wanted a song that was upbeat and not too sappy. This was the perfect combination of both," Julie says.

Still, Julie could not help but get emotional.

"Since our engagement, I had wondered whether Pete would be able to do things like walking me down the aisle and having our first dance. The fact that we were able to do both was so momentous for us."

They held each other close as loved ones stood and clapped from the edges of the dance floor.

Julie looked at Pete with a devilish grin. "Do you realize how *hot* your wife is?"

Her husband raised his eyebrows and planted another kiss on her waiting lips.

Julie's brother, who was never much for public speaking, took the microphone and told his sister and new brother-in-law how much he loved them and how special their love was.

Pete's brother then stood with a raised glass and offered the official toast for the evening. "You met the woman of your dreams on the third of July," Andrew said. "There's something special about the number 3. Pete is John Peter Frates III. You wore number 3 throughout your entire college career. You wore the number 3 at St. John's Prep, where you excelled at three sports. He graduated in 2003, John and Nancy had three kids, and he met Julie on July 3. I only have three more words to tell them—I love you."

Pete then called Nancy to the dance floor. For the traditional mother-and-son dance, they had chosen the song "Southern Cross" by Crosby, Stills & Nash. It had always been a favorite of Nancy's, but now it had special meaning for both of them. They danced gingerly as the lyrics swept across the tent—*Think about how many times I have fallen. Spirits are using me, larger voices callin'.*

Suddenly, Pete's leg gave out. He began to fall, but John and Andrew grabbed hold of him and lifted him back up. Next thing, the four of them began dancing together. Sister Jenn ran to the dance floor to join them. They created a family circle and all sang along.

Who knows love can endure. And you know it will.

———

Pete and Julie flew to the Caribbean island of Turks and Caicos for their honeymoon. They were not alone. They had decided to invite Andrew and his girlfriend with them.

"At this point, I was unable to travel anywhere with Pete alone," Julie says.

Pete had recently suffered one of many bad falls, and Julie had been unable to lift him off the floor. "I never wanted Pete to go through that again, never mind the fact that his own safety was at risk."

So the younger brother accompanied the older brother and his new bride to their tropical paradise. They rented a large two-bedroom suite, which allowed for privacy with the comfort that Andrew was close by if Pete slipped in the shower, or worse. Julie and Andrew's then girlfriend Maggie made a routine of hitting the beach in the morning while Andrew got Pete ready for the day. Soon, all four were enjoying sunshine by the pool and ocean.

"I loved going into the water with my husband," Julie says. "He was able to stand and slowly walk. It reminded me of the strong and sturdy guy he used to be. In the water he could walk around with me on his back as if he didn't have ALS. We enjoyed the normalcy of an abnormal situation."

The honeymoon was romantic for both and sometimes even farcical.

One afternoon Julie and Maggie returned to the suite to check on the boys and found Pete relaxing in the king-sized bed, while his brother was soaking in the large bathtub adjacent to the bed. The girls broke out in laughter. "It looked like Pete and Andrew were on their honeymoon." Julie recalls.

Despite Pete's physical struggles, for a brief period, at least, the couple could live in denial. They stayed in the moment, pretending to be the carefree newlyweds they so desperately wanted to be. Pete and Julie enjoyed every second of their honeymoon without dwelling on the approaching storm that would continue to alter their lives and test them in every way possible.

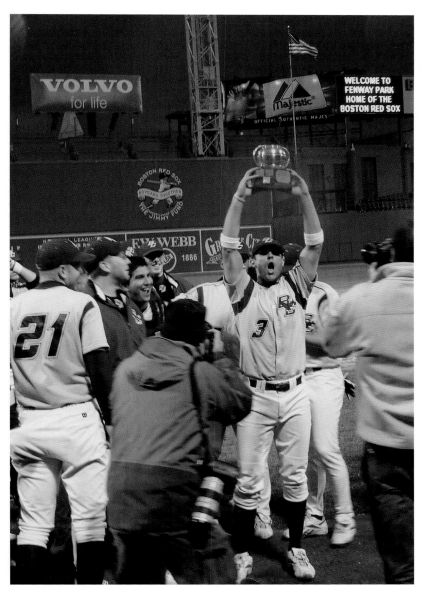

The heart of a champion. Pete Frates led the Boston
College Eagles to victory at Fenway Park, but he would
find his true mission and legacy off the playing field.
(Courtesy of Nancy Frates)

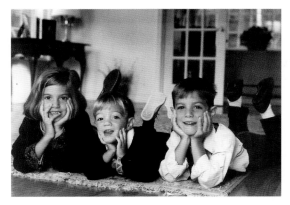

Pete's leadership skills began to emerge as a child. Seen here with his sister, Jenn, and brother, Andrew (*middle*), Pete was called "One in 10,000" by his teacher. (Courtesy of Nancy Frates)

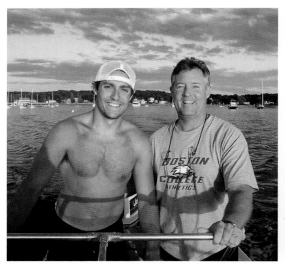

Pete's dad, John Frates, never missed one of Pete's games in high school, college, and beyond. Both share a love of sports and the ocean. (Courtesy of Nancy Frates)

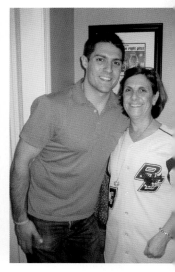

Pete's mother, Nancy Frates, battled cancer as a teenager and has proven to be a tireless advocate for her son. (Courtesy of Nancy Frates)

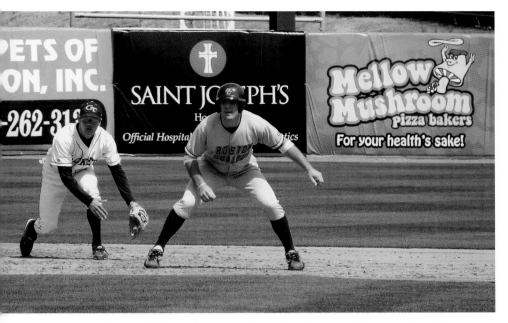

Boston College baseball coach Pete Hughes took a chance on Frates, and it paid off. Pete became one of the team's stars and was named captain during his senior year. (Courtesy of Nancy Frates)

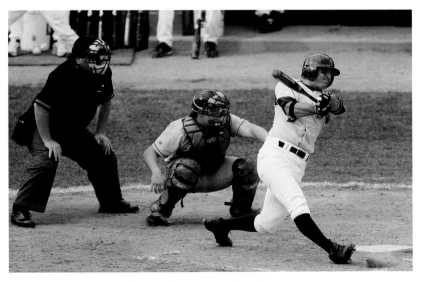

Pete was a terror on the base path, a beast at the plate, and a vacuum in the field. His physical play and focus set the tone for the BC baseball program. (Courtesy of Boston College)

Pete met his Julie just months before he was diagnosed with ALS. Described as "fearless," Julie remained by his side. (Courtesy of Nancy Frates)

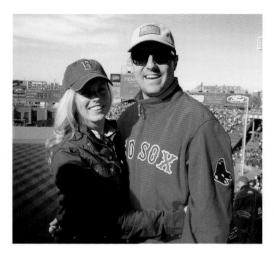

After his diagnosis, Pete found his true life's mission—to raise money for a cure for ALS. He has appeared on hundreds of television and radio programs since his diagnosis. (Courtesy of Nancy Frates)

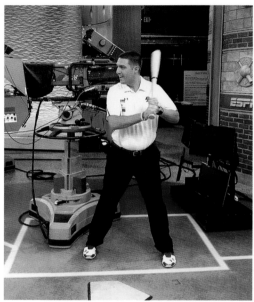

At twenty-seven years old, Pete was forced to create a bucket list of things that he and Julie wanted to do while he could still walk and breathe on his own. (Courtesy of Nancy Frates)

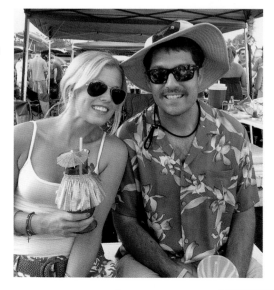

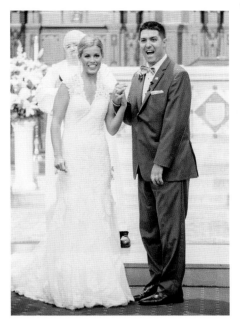

When Pete and Julie got married, his two goals were to walk her down the aisle and to have the Boston College marching band play at their wedding. He accomplished both. (Courtesy of Nancy Frates)

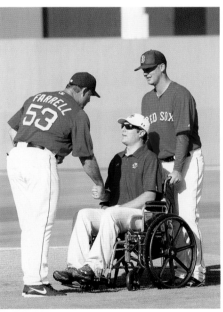

ALS ravaged Pete's body: he quickly found himself in a wheelchair and at war with his own body. (Courtesy of Nancy Frates)

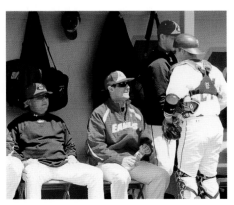

After his diagnosis, Pete was named Director of Baseball Operations at Boston College by head coach Mike Gambino. In 2016, he became only the second BC baseball player to have his number retired. (Courtesy of Boston College)

The core members of Team FrateTrain, Pete's brother, Andrew, and their sister, Jenn. All pitched in raising money and awareness for ALS, but none of them had any idea just how big their fundraising campaign would become. (Courtesy of Nancy Frates)

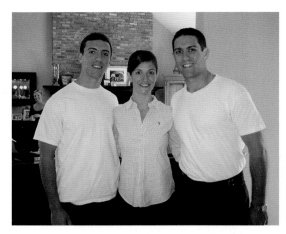

The Ice Bucket Challenge for ALS spread like wildfire in the summer of 2014 and eventually became the biggest social media campaign in history. (Courtesy of Nancy Frates)

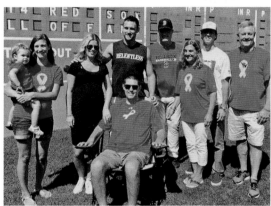

Talk Show host Oprah Winfrey doused herself with ice-cold water and then challenged Oscar-winning director Steven Spielberg to do the same. From movie studios to sandlots, supporters of all ages challenged each other, and the phenomenon grew. (YouTube)

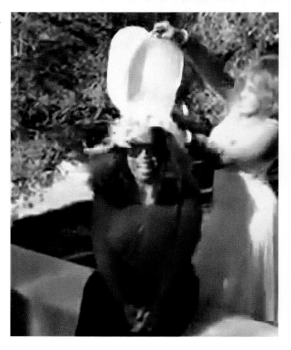

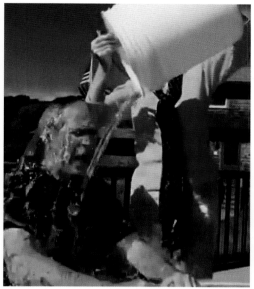

President George W. Bush took the challenge, as did President Donald Trump. President Obama did not get wet but contributed money to the cause. (YouTube)

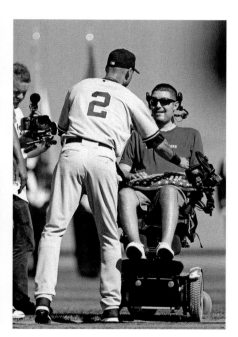

Pete Frates has done more to raise awareness for ALS than anyone since legendary New York Yankees captain Lou Gehrig. Here, Yankees captain Derek Jeter thanks Pete on behalf of the organization. (Courtesy of Nancy Frates)

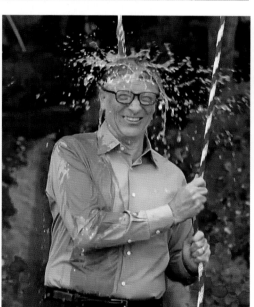

On the night of his diagnosis, Pete promised to get Microsoft founder, Bill Gates, involved in finding a cure. Gates eventually joined the cause and pulled off one of the campaign's most elaborate challenges. In total, the ALS Ice Bucket Challenge raised more than $220 million for research. (YouTube)

At the height of the hysteria surrounding the Ice Bucket Challenge, Pete and Julie celebrated another miracle, the birth of their daughter, Lucy. (Courtesy of Nancy Frates)

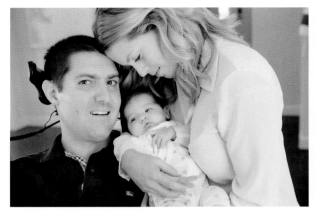

Pete sharing a tender moment with his daughter Lucy. Julie says Lucy feels most safe when she is by her father's side. (Courtesy of Nancy Frates)

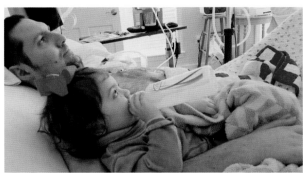

The NCAA honored Pete with its 2016 Inspiration Award, which was presented at his home in Beverly, Massachusetts. Four months later, Pete would mark his five-year anniversary as an ALS patient.

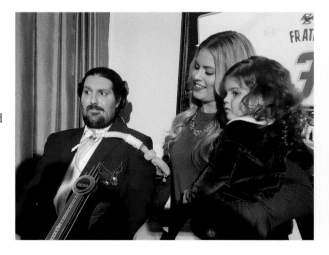

14

BACK TO THE DUGOUT

Boston College baseball coach Mike Gambino needed a spark for his team. His first two seasons had been losing efforts, and he was searching for ways to make his program competitive again, to return the baseball team to its winning ways. He called Pete at home and asked if he could take a ride to BC to talk. Pete was eager to help his friend and former coach, so John drove him from Beverly to the college campus at Chestnut Hill.

John helped Pete out of the car and assisted him as they made their way to Gambino's office. Pete was lost deep in thought as he looked around campus, remembering. He reflected back on his arrival as a freshman. He was blooming physically then and walked with confidence. He knew that the college campus would become his personal kingdom, where he would shine athletically while making hundreds of new friends along the way.

So much had changed in such a short period. Pete regained focus on the task ahead of him, which was to walk. He stepped inside Coach Gambino's office with the help of his father, and both took seats on a couch facing the coach's desk. Looking back at Pete, Gambino was shocked to see how much the disease had taken from his former star player. His once muscular build was now gone. Pete wore a short-sleeve shirt that hung off his body like it was two sizes too big.

Pete needs this as much as we do, Gambino thought.

The coach smiled. "Congratulations Pete," he said.

Pete was confused.

"Wait, what? Why are you congratulating me?" Pete asked.

"Because you are our new director of baseball operations."

Pete and John looked at each other blankly. John shrugged.

"What does the director of baseball operations do?" Pete asked.

"I don't know. I've never had one, but we'll figure it out," Gambino said. He then pointed at John and said, "And you are traveling with us, always."

It was decided that Pete would put his organizational and leadership skills to work for the program, handling travel logistics and lending his experience and knowledge to the young players. John, who had left his finance job, would be along for the ride to assist Pete. One key for Pete would be to identify "quality guys" who could serve as leaders on the team.

In his search for leaders for the coach, Pete was led back to his Lexington Blue Sox days and pointed Gambino to one of Pete's former teammates on the Intercity League squad, Chris Shaw, a six-foot, three-inch, 240-pound outfielder. Shaw swung a big bat and had a lot of raw talent that Pete suspected could blossom under the right program. He was right.

Gambino scouted Shaw, a Lexington High School graduate, and was blown away. The kid had pitched two no-hitters in high school. He was a massive left-handed power hitter and had been drafted in the twenty-sixth round by the New York Mets but was still available for Boston College. The coach loved what he saw and brought Shaw in.

It was the start of something special for Boston College, as Pete's scouting was spot-on. Shaw had an immediate impact on Gambino's squad, starting twenty-two games as a freshman and smashing six home runs. He would go on to become one of BC's most decorated players and was taken in the first round of the 2015 draft by the San Francisco Giants.

Pete and John hit the road with the team that season, living in tight quarters, sharing budget motel rooms, and eating at diners, but they had the time of their lives. John had always loved taking Pete to his games and practices when he was little, whether it was at a frigid hockey rink at five in the morning, a frosty football field on a Saturday, or a dusty baseball diamond on a scorching summer holiday. Being out on the road with BC and his son gave John a warm feeling of nostalgia and an appreciation for those carefree days when his son was just a kid.

"Just the two of them, back on the road, back with the team. I think they had a lot of fun," Julie recalls. "But I think emotionally for the both of them it was special going through that together."

Baseball acted as therapy for both John and Pete. They were able to bond as father and son all over again.

But out on the road, Pete was now firmly in charge. He took the job seriously and saw himself as a mentor to the younger players. Just as he had done as a player, Pete led by example but was often vocal. Very vocal.

At one team hotel Pete was in a wheelchair as he and a group of players waited for an elevator. A young family walked up and the elevator opened. Some of the players started to stream in, ahead of the family, incensing Pete.

"Hey, hey, guys! Let them go. Get out of the way," Pete barked.

The young players were a bit stunned at Pete's harsh tone but followed his directions. The family thanked Pete and went up the elevator. It was a small gesture that Pete made to impress on his team the importance of manners and respect for themselves and others.

He filled his time tinkering with rosters, making out hotel-room assignments, organizing team meals and meetings, and planning other logistics. There was plenty of downtime that gave John and Pete time to talk, but Pete made it clear they were not going to dwell on ALS.

At a 2013 game in North Carolina, Pete and John were staying at a Best Western, where they had a tough, but ultimately necessary, confrontation. John was struggling emotionally. He watched every day as the ballplayers all took the field healthy and with bright futures ahead of them. Why had God cursed his son with this heinous disease? John shared his feelings with Pete. The son now had to be strong for the father. Pete had cried his last tears long ago. He had questioned his faith in God and found solace in the idea that he was meant to serve a higher purpose. His was a cruel gift, but a gift just the same. He needed those around him to join in his quest or get out of his way. On unsteady feet, he stood nose to nose with John.

"Look, I've made peace with this thing," he snapped angrily. "I don't want to hear you talk about this thing anymore. I'm going to be fine. That's enough."

It was the last time they ever had a heated discussion about the disease, but it helped put John at ease that his son had accepted his fate.

"Pete was much stronger than me," John says. "He was stronger than all of us, and we drew our power from him. He was growing weaker, and yet he still felt and acted like he could run through walls."

Julie and Andrew also joined them on baseball trips. Andrew served as Pete's travel agent and handler. While Andrew pushed Pete through airports, some fellow passengers would mistakenly come up and thank Pete for his service.

"They thought he was a military veteran because he was so young," Andrew says.

Pete would make sure to correct the well-wishers, out of sheer respect for military veterans and because he wanted the opportunity to educate people about his disease. His brother would have to educate people as well.

"I would call an airline a couple days prior to our flights and make sure the airline was aware that an ALS patient would be traveling on the flight," Andrew recalls. "Most of the time, I was speaking to a customer service rep, and they had no idea what ALS was, which complicated things. I explained that Pete would need extra time down the gate, along with special instructions for the baggage crew for his wheelchair. The head piece on the power wheelchair was the most important piece on the wheelchair because this is where Pete could control the wheelchair by moving his head around with motion sensors."

Oftentimes Andrew would walk onto the tarmac and help the baggage handlers lift Pete's wheelchair onto the plane. It was thankless work, but he never complained.

"My parents, sister, and especially my brother raised me and gave me a great life," he explains. "We have a great loving family, and I saw a place where I could provide a little in return to not only Pete but to my parents and sister as well."

15

TEAM FRATE TRAIN

On each given day Pete lost a little bit more of himself, yet he refused to yield to the disease that was killing him slowly. The disease progressed through his limbs. He lost the ability to write, text with his fingers, lift a baseball bat, and drive a car. The family stood by helplessly witnessing the war that ALS was waging on his body. Fasciculations began to appear on his arms and legs. These muscle twitches or pulses under the skin amplified each battlefield in Pete's body.

"When we saw the muscles twitching and bulging in Pete's neck, we saw the horrifying reality of what was ahead," Nancy recalls.

Yet he continued his mission of ALS fund-raising and awareness and, with his family's help, he established the Pete Frates #3 Fund to help offset the high cost of his care as well as pay for the experimental drugs that he continued to take despite their apparent ineffectiveness. Pete's aunts and uncles joined the mission to build a website and handle the accounting work for the organization. Pete made sure that the number 3 appeared on the website. It was his lucky number, after all.

He had been wearing it on his uniform since he was just ten years old.

"My grandmother said I had to wear number 3 because Babe Ruth wore that," Pete recalls. "Little did I know at the time that I'd be identified more closely to the Babe's teammate Lou Gehrig."

It was time to get to work.

"The circles of Pete all started intersecting with one another," Nancy says. "This vast network of friends and family came together, and we called ourselves Team Frate Train. The train was finally on the tracks, and we were beginning to roll."

Pete named Andrew general manager of the Frate Train. Andrew created social-media platforms for the cause on Twitter and Facebook. Pete had previously given up on Facebook because he thought it had lost its coolness factor. Older people were flooding the site with photos of food, political rants, and pictures of their grandkids. But after talking it over with Andrew, Pete decided that Facebook made more sense to him now. The site had become a multigenerational platform spanning the globe and offered them the ability to reach millions of people through a click of a button. Pete wanted to begin selling T-shirts online but needed a great marketing hook. He and Andrew went out for sandwiches one day at Nick's Famous Roast Beef in Beverly and noticed photos lining the walls of the sub shop, showing patrons holding a Nick's Roast Beef bumper sticker at landmarks around the world. Team Frate Train adopted the idea. Pete and Andrew printed up red *Frates 3* T-shirts and launched a #TravelingTees social-media campaign. They recruited friends and family to pack the T-shirts on vacations and business trips, and soon Pete's message for ALS awareness and research turned up at places as far away as the Great Wall of China. Their friends also jumped in to help organize local fund-raising events, such as charity bike rides, baseball games, and bar crawls. Each endeavor was chronicled on Facebook and Twitter with the social-media hashtags #StrikeOutALS and #TeamFrateTrain. The Frates family was learning how to harness the power of social media.

While Pete's social-media presence grew, he continued to get robbed of his physical parts. He gave one of his last public speeches to a group of scientists at Biogen, Massachusetts's largest biotech company. The family was escorted to Biogen in a limousine paid for by former Boston Red Sox hurler-turned–political firebrand Curt Schilling. Pete had faced Schilling in a spring training game during his junior season at Boston College. Schilling had been a longtime supporter of the ALS Association and of Pete. He was now embroiled in an economic scandal in Rhode Island over a $75 million guaranteed loan paid out to Schilling's failed gaming company.

Despite his own troubles, Schilling came out of seclusion to join the

Frates family at Biogen. The issue at hand was not baseball, politics, or business. It was finding a cure for ALS. The drug company was finally making a return to the ALS drug market after suspending phase 3 trials of an experimental treatment. Biogen's CEO George Scangos called it "the single most negative trial I've ever seen." The trial was based on a particular drug, dexpramipexole, which had been shown to improve cellular protection of neurons under stress. It was an old-fashioned kind of trial that did not factor in the genetics of the disease, and it failed miserably. The drug trial was conducted over several years and cost more than $75 million. It also extinguished the hope of ALS patients that the world's leading experts were any closer to discovering an effective treatment. Pete was one of the patients who had participated in the trial. Now Biogen was stepping back up to the plate for another swing. This time the scientists would focus on the genetics of the neurodegenerative disease. And Pete was there to give them the ultimate locker room pep talk.

"The man upstairs has given me a plan," Pete told them. "I knew my gifts were not being used when I was an insurance salesman. Once I was diagnosed, it clicked. This is it. This is my calling. This is what I've been put here to do. The reason why there are no effective treatments for ALS, as there now are with HIV and cancer, is that we ALS patients are not around long enough to make a stink to let people know that, hey, we're here and we need a treatment and a cure. We are in a gunfight without a gun and not even a knife. We are fighting with a plastic spork."

He told the research scientists that he dreamed of the day that he could treat his symptoms with a simple pill—a pill they themselves were in the best position to produce. "From a patient, I wanted to let you know that we appreciate the serious work you do to help us."

While the researchers got down to their serious work, Pete faced a serious and precipitous decline in his health. Soon he could no longer give passionate and inspirational speeches to rally others to join his fight. He finally lost the ability to speak and was forced to use a speech-generating device and eye-gaze technology, which measures people's eye movements as they observe a computer screen.

Dr. Merit Cudkowicz had explained to the family that three primary issues could be deadly for an ALS patient—respiratory issues, malnourishment, and falls. Pete suffered a particularly bad fall while leaving a family party on Christmas Eve. John and three family members each grabbed a wheel of Pete's wheelchair and tried carrying him out of the house. The moment they reached outside, a blast of frigid air swept through, causing Pete's body to stiffen and convulse. He was propelled out of the chair and landed head first on a brick walkway. Pete suffered a deep cut to his head on impact, and blood flowed across the crevices of the bricks.

Other times both Pete's wife and his father found Pete lying helpless and alone on the floor of the adjacent apartment he shared with Julie. They quickly realized that he could never be left alone, even for a minute, ever again. The family brought in a full-time caregiver to assist with Pete's growing needs. Guy Lucien, a St. John's University graduate from New York, had previous experience as a care provider for another ALS patient.

"Guy was a godsend to us," John says. "Pete needed constant attention, with moment-to-moment adjustments to his hands, body positioning, and his ability to withstand warm and cold temperatures."

Guy, John, and Andrew worked in shifts. The professional caregiver attended to Pete during the day, while his father and brother split nights and weekends.

With Pete voiceless, his mother would have to pick up where he had left off. Nancy became the voice for Pete's mission. She hit the road with the same energy and drive she had witnessed in her son. Nancy hunted down legislators for support and spoke wherever and whenever she could gather an audience. No opportunity was too big or two small.

ALS had stripped her son of control over his body, but it could not take away his burning desire and his unwavering commitment to meet and beat any challenge—traits that he had spent years developing unknowingly in preparation for this, the fight of his life.

And now he had something else to fight for. On December 28, 2013—Pete's twenty-ninth birthday—he and Julie received the most joyous news possible. The couple was pregnant.

"It was the morning of the Plunge for Pete, an event where hundreds of people raised money for ALS by jumping into the cold Atlantic Ocean," Julie remembers. "I took a pregnancy test the day before and it was negative."

Something inside her told her that the test was wrong, so she took another the following morning. Her intuition was correct. Excited, she walked into their bedroom, where Pete was fast asleep. "Look at me," she said. "I need to tell you something."

Pete only grunted, not willing to give up his morning slumber.

Julie shook him awake. "You really need to look at me for this."

He opened his eyes and gazed at his wife. Julie had an expression of shock and anxiety on her face. "I'm pregnant," she muttered in disbelief.

Pete's eyes lit up. Instinct told him to reach for her, but his body could not move. A smile grew wide on his face. It was as if a curtain had been lifted, allowing the sunlight to shine in. Julie's doubt and fear melted away instantly. She hugged her husband as he lay on the bed.

"Congratulations, Daddy," she whispered, as she kissed his waiting lips.

———

July 4, 2014, marked the seventy-fifth anniversary of Lou Gehrig's farewell address at Yankee Stadium, where he declared himself to be "the luckiest man on the face of the earth." To commemorate the milestone, Pete was asked by MLB.com to write an article for its popular Bleacher Report on his journey from baseball star to ALS patient. He accepted the assignment, knowing that it would be the first opportunity for him to reach a national and international audience.

"I once prided myself on my strong hands," he wrote. "They helped me grip the bat, fire the barrel through the zone and squeeze a fly ball safely into my outfield mitt. Today, they are unable to type this very story, as I depend on eye-tracking technology to deliver the message that my sturdy voice and fingers once did."

Pete described the overwhelming challenge faced by ALS patients and researchers every day. "What if you woke up today and someone told you that you have two to five years to live? How would you handle the news? What if they told you that during those two to five years you would lose control of your extremities and your ability to speak, eat and breathe?"

His words were unforgiving, and, through that honesty, he had the ability to place the reader in his wheelchair and offer them a perspective that they may not have experienced before. While Lou Gehrig had shown dignity in fighting his disease with quiet courage, Pete was in-your-face, showing the public the pain and indignity patients like him suffered every day. Pete was also willing to call out Major League Baseball for its lack of effort in finding a cure for ALS.

"MLB as a whole has shouldered some of this burden, and rightfully so," he wrote. "The fact is, the illness bears one of its legends' names, and the league has both the audience and the power to make change."

While Gehrig was soft-spoken and private, Pete was a firebrand, criticizing anyone or any organization who believed that since ALS affected a relatively small portion of the population, it was a disease not worth fighting for or, in this case, fighting against. Their personalities and styles differed greatly, but Pete still found his inspiration from the Iron Horse of a bygone era. "I have a poster of his [Gehrig's] speech on the wall of my garage," Pete wrote. "It is the last thing I see when I leave the house. I use his words to help me attack the day and keep up the fight against the beast that is ALS."

The editors at MLB.com had expected that Pete's story might trigger a bump in visits to their website, but they never imagined the outpouring of interest generated by the article. The story was read by 324,000 people around the world.

With a gut-wrenching yet simple online article, Pete had increased awareness for the disease to a level never seen before. Yet awareness did not translate to money. People were still donating to causes elsewhere.

"I don't get it," Nancy told John in frustration. "As a family, we have dedicated our lives to caring for Pete and to raising funds to find a cure. We've exhausted every avenue, and still we feel that we are at the base of the mountain with a huge climb ahead of us. I don't know what else we can do."

Almost a year to the day after Pete's ALS diagnosis in 2012, another young man had received similar startling news from his own doctors. A couple hundred miles away, in Yonkers, New York, Pat Quinn had just celebrated his thirtieth birthday when an unusual series of aches and numbness led him to seek medical help. Pat suspected that he may have been stricken with Lyme disease and was stunned when doctors explained the source of his affliction. "I thought it was a disease that struck elderly people," he recalled. "I was in the prime of my life."

Like Pete, Pat was not going to "go gentle into that good night." Instead, he would "rage against the dying of the light." Just as Pete had done, Quinn used the best tool available to him and took his fight to the Internet in search of answers, help, or anything to offer him hope.

He found that hope when he stumbled across Pete's website. Pat read about Pete and his Plunge for Pete fund-raisers, saw how organized his awareness and fund-raising campaign was, and wanted to learn. Pete became an immediate mentor to Pat, long before they had even communicated with each other.

Pat showed his girlfriend, Jennifer Flynn, Pete's website and told her, "This is how we have to do it."

"You need to get in touch with this guy," she told him.

Pat got to the task of composing an e-mail to Pete, introducing himself and seeking to partner up in the fight against the disease that was consuming both young men. But Pat was a bit gun-shy and delayed sending the e-mail.

For weeks.

Two months went by, and despite Jennifer's daily reminders Pat did not send the e-mail. One day they were riding in the car, and Jen asked him, "Did you send that e-mail yet to Pete Frates?"

"No," Pat answered sheepishly.

She pulled the car over, grabbed his phone, looked into Pat's e-mail, and fired off an updated missive to Pete that would alter the course of both of their lives.

Below is the e-mail message, as it was sent to the general contact form on Pete's website:

Good afternoon,

My name is Pat Quinn and I am from Yonkers, NY. I was diagnosed with ALS *this past March and am 30 years old. It has been truly inspiring coming across Pete's page and seeing all that Pete has done in such little time. I really hope I can begin to do some of the things Pete has been able to do soon. I want to be the advocate he is and fight this thing with everything I got.*

The reason for the email today is I am coming up to MA next week to visit ALSTDI *(*ALS *Therapy Development Institute). I know this is in Cambridge and a place Pete has been affiliated with. I saw his speech at the Gala last year and like I stated before, I have been*

truly inspired by Pete. His motivation and determination are quali-
ties I believe I possess, as well, and look to develop into a great force
in this fight for awareness, treatments, and eventually a cure. Sorry
I got sidetracked, but again the email was to see if Pete would be in
the Cambridge/Boston area on Friday, I would love the opportunity
to meet him after I tour TDI. *I think we have a lot in common and*
it would be an honor.

Please let me know if this would be possible. If not, I hope to hear
he will be attending the Gala this year at TDI. *I believe I will be in*
attendance.

Have a happy 4th and I appreciate your time.
Thanks,
Patrick Quinn
P.S. I am not a crazy Yankee fan or anything, but I do root for
them. LOL

It was that last sentence that caught Pete's eye. A baseball fan with a sense of humor. Now that was something Pete could relate to. Pete became Pat's mentor, just as Steve Gleason had become Pete's a year earlier when Pete was diagnosed. Pete wanted to pay it forward, and in Pat he saw many of the same characteristics of himself: determination, grit, drive, and passion. There was also a kinship in the fact that they were both much younger than the average ALS patient.

When Pat Quinn and his girlfriend visited Boston, they met with Pete and Julie at a tavern in Charlestown.

"Immediately upon meeting them, I knew we would have a connec-tion," Julie says. "Pat and Jen were so warm and funny and honestly reminded me of Pete and me."

Like the Frates, Pat and his girlfriend fell in love hard and fast, and Jen made the choice to stay with Pat after his diagnosis, knowing it was not going to be easy. That day at the tavern, Pat asked Pete question after question about living with the disease and about fighting back.

"I still haven't told everyone about my diagnosis," Pat told them.

Pete was stunned. It had been more than two months since Pat received the life-changing news that he had ALS, and he had told no one but his girlfriend and a few family members.

"That's totally unacceptable," Pete replied. "You cannot go through this alone. You need to assemble all of your networks to be in your corner."

Pete told Pat flatly that there would be no hope for a cure if the afflicted did not speak up, if the afflicted did not get angry. Pete was nearly one year further progressed into the disease, and he offered to be Pat's guide through the many challenges to come, those known and those unknown.

"Pat needed Pete's mentorship, but Pete needed Pat as well," Julie says. "The relationship gave Pete purpose. He was no longer on the receiving end of someone else's support. Pete was now able to help someone else in such a profound way."

Julie and Pete counseled Pat and Jennifer about how to build their team, not only to raise awareness of ALS, but to support the soon-to-escalate cost of Pat's care. Pat was unaware of the astronomical cost of care, and Pete and Julie helped the young couple set up Pat's foundation, Quinn for the Win.

The two men forged a close friendship, bound by grueling shared experiences and a determination to find a cure. With guidance from his mentor, Pat grew to become a vocal advocate in the ALS community and soon came in contact with other families stuck in the same unimaginable situation, each fighting their own battles and claiming their own small victories amid crushing defeats. One ALS patient, Anthony Senerchia of Pelham, New York, had surpassed his life expectancy by living with the disease for eleven years and earning the admiration of friends, family, and total strangers alike.

It was a seemingly mundane show of support for Senerchia from a semifamous relative that would provide the spark for Pete's mission to alter the course of ALS and change the world. Professional golfer Chris Kennedy, a cousin of Senerchia's wife, Jeanette, filled a bucket with ice water and dumped it on his head as a friend filmed the stunt with his cell phone. Standing in the backyard of his Florida home, Kennedy held a small plastic bucket with both hands and challenged Jeanette and two others to do the same. "You have twenty-four hours to respond, or you're gonna donate a hundred dollars to the ALS Foundation," Kennedy said before dousing himself. "Good luck, guys."

It was a stunt other pro golfers had done occasionally as a way to raise money and awareness for various charities. Participants had a choice to douse themselves with ice cold water or send money to a particular charity. Normally, those accepting the challenge did both. Jeanette saw the video pop up on her Facebook news feed and laughed.

"You have to be kidding me," she told Kennedy. "I'm not gonna do it. I'll just donate a hundred dollars to ALS instead."

Kennedy pleaded with his cousin to accept his challenge, which she did a day later, as her six-year-old daughter filmed her in the front of their New York home. The date was July 16, 2014.

Jeanette Senerchia challenged two cousins and a friend—passing it along like a cyber chain letter—and one of the people she tagged in the video happened to also be a Facebook friend of Pat Quinn. Pat and his family made some similar videos of their own, one of which he tagged Pete in, hoping his ALS mentor would see it. The videos were fun, but no one could have predicted what Pete was about to make happen.

16

THE ICE BUCKET CHALLENGE

The first video flashed on Pete's computer screen. He watched, smiled, and an idea began to form. "This is exactly what we've been waiting for," Pete thought immediately. "I've been preaching, calling for mobilization and the opportunity to raise money to fight ALS on a mass scale. I've been developing and building a large and powerful network of supporters and influencers for this very reason."

He watched it again. And again. And he found some others. The Ice Bucket Challenge had not yet been connected officially to ALS, but Pete saw this as the vehicle to change the course of the disease forever. He started researching the Ice Bucket Challenge. He was a social-media dynamo who had already built up a large network of followers on Facebook and Twitter who were supporting his ALS fight every day and helping make his Pete Frates #3 Fund a regional success story. When he saw that the challenge had not yet been officially tied to any particular charity, he decided it was time he and his army of ALS warriors claim it as their own.

He spelled out words furiously with his eye gazer and called Julie and Nancy in from the backyard. "We are going to start seeing people pouring ice water over their heads," he told them. "We've been building momentum for this disease. Here it is. This is it!"

Nancy had no idea what her son was talking about.

"Quick, get on your computers and start liking and sharing every one of these videos you see on our Team Frate Train home page on Facebook,"

Pete ordered. "Comment on everything. Please say, 'Thank you. Thank you for joining us in this fight.'"

Andrew had recently gone back to work at their alma mater St. John's Prep. He was attending a conference at the University of Vermont and jumped into action to help his brother. He went to a gas station and bought a bag of ice, grabbed a dirty trash can from his hotel room and performed the stunt outside in the pouring rain. He challenged his father in the video and then called him.

"You need to grab ice, put it in a bucket, and dump water over your head," Andrew told him. "Challenge three people, Pete's friends Tommy Haugh and Mike Budreau and a person of your choice. Make sure you tag them on Facebook. This is very important to do it within twenty-four hours!"

John rushed into the backyard with Pete and caregiver Guy Lucien. He dumped a bag of ice and water in an old wheelbarrow and lay down on the patio. Lucien lifted the end of the wheelbarrow and poured the ice water on Pete's dad with glee. The old wheelbarrow had special meaning for John and Pete. As a boy, Pete had used it to help his dad on backyard gardening projects. The hard work helped Pete build his muscles. After he had been hit by that pitch in 2011, Pete was helping John unload a truck full of topsoil and pushed the wheelbarrow as he had always done. But this time it slipped out of his left hand, and the topsoil spilled onto the driveway. "When are you gonna get that wrist checked?" John asked. It was an ominous sign of the trouble ahead. Now the wheelbarrow was being used to exorcize old demons.

For the first twenty-four hours, Nancy, Julie, and John barely left their seats at the kitchen table. The videos started coming in once every half hour. Soon they were coming in every half second. They liked, tagged, commented, and shared hundreds of videos that came pouring in. Pete served as the field general, barking orders through his computer and offering words of encouragement to his troops.

He then e-mailed every professional athlete, politician, and influencer he knew and urged them all to join his team.

Most of Pete's family and friends had their own Facebook accounts, but his uncle Dave Cloyd, who managed his website, did not. Uncle Dave was not on social media and had not seen any of the videos, so he had no idea why he kept getting notification after notification that people were clicking onto Pete's website. It was a flurry of activity that the uncle could not explain, so he immediately texted Pete's mother.

"Nancy, what the hell is going on?" he asked. "Pete's website is blowing up!"

Nancy's thoughts drifted back to the panel of frustrated ALS experts who, despite their backgrounds, did not seem to know how to accomplish the goal of eradicating this deadly disease once and for all.

The Ice Bucket Challenge had had been around for some time, and people had used it to raise money for a wide range of causes. But no charity had truly owned it. Through two years of outreach and advocacy for ALS, the Frates family had built a vast network of supporters throughout the country. It was time to harness all that positive energy and mobilize an army for good. And Facebook was their Trojan horse.

"We are planting our flag for ALS with this," Pete told his parents through his mechanical device. "This is what we have been waiting for. This is it."

Nancy agreed. "The disease needs more funding," she said. "We need the brightest medical researchers to join the fight, and the only way to do that is to raise more money. We need ice, a bucket, and everyone to donate a hundred to the cause."

On July 31, 2014, Pete made his first Ice Bucket Challenge video, but it actually involved no water and a different type of ice: rapper Vanilla Ice. Because Pete's body was ultrasensitive to hot and cold temperatures, he opted not to dump freezing water over his head and instead posted a video of himself nodding along and smiling in front of the Vanilla Ice video for the song "Ice Ice Baby." He tagged all sorts of celebrities, including New England Patriots stars Tom Brady and Julian Edelman; Pete's BC pal Matt Ryan of the Atlanta Falcons; Red Sox player Will Middlebrooks; Sox owner John Henry; Howard Stern, a writer for the popular sports site Barstool Sports; and Boston sports talk show hosts Fred Toucher and Rich Shertenlieb.

"So I am nominating myself for the #icebucketchallenge cuz I can. . . . Ice water and ALS are a bad mix, so I got my friend Rob Van Winkle (aka

Vanilla Ice) to help me out," Pete wrote in the post. He told them all, "You have 24 hours to dump a bucket of ice over your head" and added the hashtags #StrikeOutALS and #QuinnForTheWin.

Meanwhile, Nancy sat down with other members of Team Frate Train and devised a strategy to monetize Pete's website like never before. There was a donation button on Pete's website. The trust had been established to help pay for the ballooning costs of Pete's health care. The family decided to add other charity organizations to Pete's home page. They listed four other places to donate, with detailed descriptions of their missions and a link to their home pages. They added the ALS Foundation, Compassionate Care ALS, the Angel Fund, and the ALS Therapy Development Institute.

"A very conscious decision was made not to send a directive to donate to any one organization," Nancy recalls. "We just kept saying the words 'ALS' and let people educate themselves and choose where they wanted their money to go."

She then ran to the backyard and performed the Ice Bucket Challenge herself.

Since Pete's diagnosis, the family had used #StrikeOutALS on all social-media posts. Now Pete gave the order to add two more hashtags—#ALS IceBucketChallenge and #IceBucketChallenge. The challenge quickly spread through their hometown of Beverly, Massachusetts, then to Boston and beyond.

Matt Ryan, an emerging National Football League star at the time, was among the first major celebrities to answer the call on a national level. Ryan had met Pete during their freshmen orientation at BC, and the two became fast friends. Wearing his practice jersey and shorts, Ryan, a future NFL MVP stood on the field of the Falcons' Georgia practice facility, filled a Gatorade bucket with ice, and poured it over his head before challenging three teammates to do the same. Another BC football legend, Doug Flutie, also supported Pete with a splash of his own. Other NFL stars, such as Green Bay Packers quarterback Aaron Rodgers and Denver Broncos legend Peyton Manning, followed. The staggering social-media followings of each athlete fueled the cyber wildfire, as video after video went viral.

New York Yankees captain Derek Jeter took the challenge in the locker room at Yankee Stadium, where the legend of Lou Gehrig had been born nearly a hundred years before. Jeter acknowledged the former team captain, who was now a worldwide symbol for ALS, and also tipped his proverbial cap to Pete. "[Pete] was the former captain of the Boston College baseball team who was the whole inspiration behind this Ice Bucket Challenge," Jeter said, before being doused with a bucket filled with icy water. Jeter then passed the challenge along to another sports icon, Chicago Bulls Hall of Famer Michael Jordan. Air Jordan accepted the challenge.

Pat Quinn appeared at a Chicago White Sox game and talked about how it went from a lighthearted game among friends to the viral sensation, thanks to his friend Pete. "It got up to Boston, and it just caught fire. . . . It's out of control," Quinn told the MLB Network. "The Ice Bucket Challenge is fun. That's the whole reason it caught on. But you have to get behind the cause."

The videos kept coming. But now they also included donations to fund ALS research. Pete's website and his Facebook and Twitter pages exploded. The family's Beverly home was transformed into a command center for the viral sensation, now known as the Ice Bucket Challenge for ALS.

People young and old and from all over began to send cards and letters to the Frates home. Many of the envelopes were stuffed with donations, while others offered words of support.

Letters came from family friends: "Dear Nancy and John, I cannot begin to know how difficult each day is for the both of you, but I can tell you that your courage, strength and utter devotion to your children has been an inspiration to me and countless others," wrote Leigh Santer of Mansfield, Massachusetts.

Letters came from caring strangers: "All the best to Pete and his family in this incredible struggle and fight with ALS. Thank you for your courage," wrote Jenny Buchar of Park City, Utah.

Letters came from those who understood the family's struggle: "From one fighter to another. I beat cancer three years ago. You are an inspiration telling your story," wrote Sarah Bondarev of Wichita, Kansas.

"I did not take the Ice Bucket Challenge," wrote Mark and Molly Howe, of Michigantown, Indiana. "But I want to donate in memory of Jim Lipinski, a dear friend who passed away years ago from complications of Lou Gehrig's disease. RIP Jim."

Donations came from the folks at the Lighthouse Cove Tiki Bar in Pompano Beach, Florida, who held a nonstop twenty-four-hour Ice Bucket Challenge. They came from the Peoria Hash House Harriers in Illinois, a self-proclaimed drinking group with a running problem. They came from businesses and colleges across the country. They came from churches with envelopes stuffed with cash and prayer cards.

Letters and donations came from the oldest among us: "My name is Bea Beer," wrote a woman in Gainesville, Florida. "I am 88-years-old and I did the Ice Bucket Challenge with my daughter. I am happy to support ALS and Pete Frates!"

They came from the children who sent Pete their drawings of baseballs, hearts, and sunrises: Taryn Francel, an elementary school teacher from El Cajon, California, got her students to write letters to Pete and his family.

"I will do anything to raise money for ALS and my grandma," wrote a student named Taylor. "She had ALS and then she died."

"I know you can get through this," wrote a girl named Tirra. "I believe you are stronger than you think. I know you might feel like you can't do much, but you can do great things. I believe in you and you can get better."

Television reporters began to show up to the Frates house unannounced. The family's answering machine overflowed with requests for radio interviews from all over the world. A reporter from NHL.com phoned John Frates from Montreal after seeing the league's top player take the challenge.

"Why is Sidney Crosby dumping water on his head and shouting Pete's name?" the reporter asked. "As Sidney goes, so goes the nation." Canadians took their lead from the Pittsburgh Penguins superstar and ultimately donated $17 million to the cause.

Friends jumped in to help, including a next-door neighbor who knocked on the door with a stack of pizzas. "I thought you might need food in here," he said, pointing to his special delivery of hot pizza pies.

Julie was now nine months pregnant and just weeks from delivering the couple's child. She looked out the front window of their home to see an army of reporters camped outside. "My hormones are raging, and I don't think I can handle it all," she told Pete.

"We'll get through it, babe," he replied using his eye gazer. "This is going to change the course of ALS forever." Pete was right. The acronym ALS was now on everyone's lips like never before in history, and it was nearly impossible to keep up with it all, as adults and kids from across the United States began to mobilize and recruit others to the cause.

The phenomenon was capturing the world's attention, spreading across the globe via Facebook and Twitter in mere days, as seemingly everyone on the planet got in on the fun. Singer-actor Justin Timberlake was among the first international superstars to post a video.

"J. T. here," he said, leaning into the camera, wearing a Pink Floyd T-shirt and baseball cap. "I am accepting the ALS Ice Bucket Challenge. . . . I am gonna pass this on and challenge Jimmy Fallon, Steve Higgins, and The Roots from *Fallon Tonight*. Here we go."

Timberlake then joined more than a dozen friends and fans in hoisting ice-cold buckets of water over their own heads. Fallon, a native of New Hampshire, quickly accepted the challenge, as did Oprah Winfrey.

"In the name of ALS, I accept this challenge," said the talk show queen. "Steven Spielberg, I challenge you next. I know where you live." The bucket was lifted and the ice-cold water cascaded down over the entertainment icon. Oprah let out an ear-piercing scream. Clearly, she was not prepared for the frigid sensation, but she proved to be a great sport for a greater cause.

Spielberg, the Oscar-winning director, followed suit, as more and more celebrities brought more and more attention and donations to the Frates family and ALS organizations everywhere.

"I'm gonna take the challenge and make a donation," said fellow Oscar-winner Ben Affleck, a native of Cambridge, Massachusetts, as he stood in front of the pool at his Los Angeles–area home. He nominated other people who he said looked "good" in a wet T-shirt, including pals Matt Damon and Jimmy Kimmel and actor Jennifer Garner, Affleck's wife. Garner poured the bucket on Affleck's head, and he then grabbed her and tossed her into the pool, as their children laughed uncontrollably.

Members of Pearl Jam, Pete's favorite band, poured cold ice water on their heads after being challenged by Steve Gleason, who had built up a friendship with the Seattle super group. Lead singer Eddie Vedder performed the challenge on a beach in Seattle. Vedder then challenged actor Tim Robbins, Bruce Springsteen, and, at his young daughters' request, Niall Horan from pop band One Direction. Gleason could hardly believe what was happening.

"We see thousands of people participating," the ex-NFL player said. "It's raised more awareness of the disease than anything in the history of ALS since Lou Gehrig's announcement seventy-five years ago." But, he added, "Contrary to what Lou Gehrig said, ALS patients are not in any way lucky. It's a silent, brutal, and until now an anonymous death. There is still no treatment or cure."

The list of A-list celebrities participating in the viral sensation continued to grow. Kim Kardashian, Lady Gaga, Taylor Swift, Tom Cruise, Leonardo DiCaprio, Rihanna, Robert Downey Jr., and dozens more joined Pete's army. His fellow athletes also felt the chill, including NBA stars Lebron James and Kevin Durant; the entire squads of the Boston Red Sox, New England Patriots, and New York Jets; and—the most spectacular—NHL player Paul Bissonnette, who doused glacier water from a helicopter onto his head while standing atop a mountain in a Speedo. The challenges grew more widespread and more elaborate and outlandish. And the money, like the ice water, poured in.

Pete demanded to know every possible detail about how widespread the Ice Bucket Challenge had become and, more important, how much money it was generating. Each morning Nancy spoke with Lynn Aaronson, the executive director of the ALS Association's Massachusetts chapter, who provided her with donation numbers statewide and on a national level. Aaronson had recently done the challenge herself and recruited her own staff to like and share videos on social media. Aaronson's office was overwhelmed with hundred-dollar donations that quickly added up. The ALS Association received $1 million overnight and then a whopping $13 million in a twenty-four-hour period. In Aaronson's office alone, it took three staffers nearly an hour each morning just to open all the mail.

Nancy called down to the ALS Association Office in Washington, DC, to check on donations. She gave her name and was transferred to the director of marketing, Carrie Munk.

"We all know who you are," Munk told Nancy. "You have completely turned our world upside down."

The ALS Association was not prepared for the social-media onslaught. In just a few short weeks, the organization had attracted 2.5 million more donors to its cause. The organization's website was not optimized to handle the amount of new traffic and the millions of donations coming in minute by minute. Carrie Munk recruited Brian Frederick from the public relations firm Porter Novelli to handle the growing media requests and letters from people from around the world about the Ice Bucket Challenge.

"There were stacks and stacks of mail," Frederick says. "There was also an overwhelming amount of e-mail that had to be responded to. It burned a lot of folks here out. It was a great challenge for our folks, though. It's easy to get down on yourselves and distraught battling this disease, but Pete is an inspiration to everyone that meets him, and he strengthens the resolve of all of us who continue to fight this battle."

The campaign was also wearing out Pete's pregnant wife. "I kept waking up every morning, thinking, 'Well, it's gotta be over now,'" remembers Julie.

But instead, it showed no signs of slowing down—quite the opposite. The Ice Bucket Challenge traveled from the United States to Canada first, then spread to Europe, Australia, and other parts of the world. Even redemption nuns in Dublin, Ireland, felt compelled to drench their habits. "Jesus, I pray for you," one of the nuns said cheerfully, as her fellow sisters poured tiny buckets of cold water down on them. The nuns screamed, clapped, and giggled their way through the ordeal, chanting "Oh, Lord," with thick Irish brogues. That video alone received more than 180,000 views on YouTube.

Every day provided a new chapter for Nancy. For her, one of the most touching moments came from Max Kennedy, son of the late Robert F. Kennedy. He sent her an e-mail with a video attached: "I want to thank you for the great work you are doing on behalf of everyone with ALS, but also every human being for giving us a chance to participate," Kennedy wrote. "My mother [Ethel Kennedy] is 86-years-old and a group of her children and grandchildren got together and challenged my mom. . . . So many amazing videos have been made as part of this challenge, but I thought, particularly because you are also a large Irish Catholic Boston family that you would find this fun." In the video, family matriarch Ethel Kennedy challenged President Barack Obama himself.

President Obama declined Ethel Kennedy's challenge and instead opted to donate a hundred dollars for ALS research. His predecessor, former president George W. Bush, posted a video thanking all those who challenged him, including his daughter Jenna Bush and NFL coach Jim Harbaugh and golf champion Rory McIlroy. "I do not think it's presidential for me to be splashed with ice water, so I'm simply going to write you a check," President Bush said in the video. Seconds later former First Lady Laura Bush entered the frame with a bucket and let go, drenching the former commander in chief. Standing by her soaked husband, a perfectly quaffed Mrs. Bush had her own message for the American people: "That check is from me. I didn't want to ruin my hairstyle."

Even future U.S. president Donald Trump took the challenge, with tongue planted firmly in cheek. High atop Trump Tower, flanked by Miss Universe and Miss USA, Trump sat on a stool in his customary dark suit with red tie and spoke into the camera. "Everybody's going crazy over this thing," Trump said about the Ice Bucket Challenge. "I guess they want to see whether or not it's my real hair, which it is." The water came down, and the hair fell matted and wet over his forehead. Trump then nominated his sons and President Obama, the man he would eventually succeed in the White House.

Pete, Julie, and their family continued to watch, as the videos and donations flooded in. One particular video brought the Frates family's efforts full circle.

"I'm gonna convince philanthropists like Bill Gates to get involved," Pete had promised his distraught family members on the very day of his diagnosis during that powerful kitchen-table rally speech. On August 15, 2014, the Microsoft mogul *did* get involved. Answering a challenge laid down by Facebook founder Mark Zuckerberg, Gates said that he was glad to give to ALS, as it was a great cause. He went on to say that he also wanted to accept the challenge and "do it better than it had been done before."

In an elaborately produced video, the billionaire is shown devising and welding a steel contraption to hold an ice bucket. "I'm here, joining the people who are bringing attention to Lou Gehrig's disease by taking the ALS Ice Bucket Challenge." Gates said. After challenging three more people, including tech billionaire Elon Musk and American Idol host Ryan Seacrest, Gates yanked on a rope, pulling down a bucketful of ice water on his head.

Upon seeing this video, Nancy broke out in tears. "[Pete] told us that he'd get Bill Gates involved in raising money and awareness for this disease, and that's exactly what he did," Nancy says.

Pete was also overwhelmed. This was validation for two years of the most arduous human struggle imaginable. During each step of this difficult journey—when pain shot through his body, when he was lying on the floor helpless and bloodied, when the disease had stripped him of his dignity—he found solace and comfort in the belief that eventually he would reach a philanthropist as powerful as Bill Gates with his mission.

Now he had accomplished just that.

Pete had believed in visualization. If you think about it, if you dream it, and, most important, if you work harder than anyone else thought possible, you can do it.

With the Bill Gates's video, Pete had reached his personal summit, and although the view was breathtaking, he realized that his work was far from done. "Mission accomplished," Pete told his family. "But there are still more mountains to climb."

The world had rallied around Pete, Pat Quinn, Anthony Senerchia, and ALS patients and their families. It was time for Pete to acknowledge their compassion and generosity in the only way he knew how. John, Nancy, Andrew, Julie, Jenn, and her husband, Dan, piled into a van and drove down to Fenway Park. It was the site of Pete's greatest baseball moment, when he had hit that home run during the Beanpot Tournament so many years before. That triumph though, was infinitely small compared to what he, his family, and others had just accomplished. Pete was wheeled out to the outfield of his favorite ballpark. A bucket was filled. Julie, pregnant and healthy, grabbed the bucket with both hands.

"Are you ready for this?" she asked.

A smile spread across her husband's face. He had been ready for this his whole life. He had been ready for an opportunity to make a difference. He had been ready for a chance to change the world. Julie lifted the bucket of ice water and poured it over the head of her husband, her life partner, and her champion. Miracles can happen.

The month of August 2014 ended with another miracle. Julie accomplished a mission of her own by giving birth to their daughter, Lucy Fitzgerald Frates. The excitement and enthusiasm about what they had achieved with the Ice Bucket Challenge followed the couple into the maternity ward. "Pete and I arrived at the hospital, and I was having contractions every five minutes and doubling over in pain," Julie recalls.

"People kept coming up to us, saying, 'Oh my God, you're the guy behind the Ice Bucket Challenge!'"

Pete stopped and said hello to the well-wishers.

"Meanwhile, I'm actively in labor," Julie laughs. "I'm thinking, 'Can't these people see what's going on here?'"

They entered the delivery room together. The doctor and nurses came in and began to coach Julie through the delivery. Pete watched as his beautiful wife was about to give him the ultimate gift.

The gift of life.

Another small miracle then took place.

Pete began straining his vocal chords. He had not spoken a word in several months. But he knew that Julie needed to hear his voice. The words came slow and softly. But the words came.

"Go, babe," he said using every ounce of his strength. "You got this."

The nurses at Julie's bedside heard only muffled sounds and could not understand what Pete was trying to say. Julie knew exactly what the man she loved more than anything in the world was telling her. A sense of calm washed over her at that moment. "He gave me the strength and support I needed to bring our baby into the world," she remembers.

Baby Lucy weighed in at seven pounds, eight ounces, and attached herself to her stricken father right away, as Julie placed the infant gently on her husband's chest. Pete could feel his daughter's tiny heart beating against his own, and she could feel his.

"Fatherhood means everything to me," Pete said at the time through his computer-generated voice. "It is my driving force to keep battling every day so that one day I can see Lucy grow into a wonderful, beautiful woman."

17

THE LONG RUN

A few short months after the Ice Bucket Challenge, officials at Facebook invited Nancy; Pat Quinn and his wife, Jen; and Jeanette and Anthony Senerchia to a meeting at their offices in New York City. These were the three families responsible for the largest fund-raising drive in the history of social media. The families were escorted into the building and led to a boardroom, where a group of Facebook's top analysts were waiting. They took their seats around a long conference table, as their attention was drawn to a large wall screen, where Facebook's then chief information officer, Tim Campos, appeared. Campos wanted to show the families the massive global reach of their efforts.

"This is the biggest thing to have ever happened to our platform," Campos said. "We would like to share with you the following metrics. Your efforts were jaw dropping. Seventeen million videos were posted on Facebook. Our repetitive-use statistics show that each user watched each Ice Bucket Challenge video between ten and fifteen times. The videos were watched by 440 million people in 150 countries around the world. The ALS Ice Bucket Challenge videos were viewed more than 10 billion times."

Nancy felt her own jaw drop, as she tried to wrap her head around that last number.

Ten Billion.

A map appeared on the screen, as Facebook executives tracked the social-media campaign's movement across the globe. It started in the

United States but exploded when it got to Boston, thanks to Pete's network of supporters. From there it shot over to Canada, then Ireland, where Pat Quinn has relatives and where the Boston College brand is strong. Then the Ice Bucket Challenge traveled to Germany, where Pete had collected a wide group of friends while playing baseball for the Hamburg Stealers, and beyond. In just two short months, from July to August 2014, the ALS Ice Bucket Challenge had become the most successful social-media campaign in the history of the world, touching nearly every corner of the earth from working-class families to the rich and famous. The statistics across other social-media platforms were equally impressive. On Twitter, the Ice Bucket Challenge generated 15.5 million mentions over July and August 2014. On Instagram 3.7 million videos were uploaded with #ALSIceBucketChallenge or #IceBucketChallenge. A full 6.2 million videos were uploaded on YouTube with Bill Gates's Ice Bucket Challenge proving most popular at nearly 12 million views. Google later reported that ALS was its number-one searched topic in its "what is" category for 2014.

Pete felt that he was no longer bound by his motorized wheelchair. Instead, he had traveled the globe, with the help of modern technology, to bring his mission to the masses. ALS was no longer a seldom discussed and acknowledged disease. It had become one of the most commonly known afflictions in the world. There was hope.

And, finally, there was the funding to fight it and find a cure. Pete had mobilized a global army for good, and millions paid it forward by sharing large sums or what little they had. By the end of 2014, the ALS Association had raised $160 million from the awareness brought by the Ice Bucket Challenge.

That number has ballooned to more than $220 million today.

The hundreds of millions of dollars donated by people from around the world are currently being spent on five medical areas: gene discovery, disease-model development, clinical trials, drug development, and patient care. Many experts believe there will be a treatment to curb the progression of ALS within five years.

Over the next year Pete, Nancy, and the family were showered with awards honoring their historic work in the funding fight for ALS research. Pete was named Inspiration of the Year by *Sports Illustrated*. He was also a top-twenty nominee for *Time* magazine's Person of the Year honor in 2015.

New England Patriots owner Robert Kraft honored Pete on his birthday and led fans at a sold-out Patriots game at Gillette Stadium in a chorus of the birthday song for the ALS warrior. The Red Sox, Pete's favorite team, signed him to a ceremonial player contract. Despite Pete's new-found celebrity, he never let all the attention get to his head. His message and mission remained clear. The more money spent on research, the greater likelihood that scientists would be able to help those suffering from ALS lead healthier and longer lives and to eradicate this terrible disease from the earth once and for all.

But there would be more hardships on the way. The Frates family was still reeling from the death of twenty-seven-year-old Corey Griffin, a former Boston College hockey player and close friend of Pete's who had been instrumental in the Ice Bucket Challenge. In August 2014 Griffin had raised approximately $100,000 dollars to fight ALS. He had organized the largest Ice Bucket Challenge in the parking lot of a telecommunications firm in Quincy, Massachusetts, where 1,200 people took part. He texted Pete moments after with the exciting news. Just hours later Griffin visited the island of Nantucket, where he took a late-night celebratory dive off a building on the wharf into the dark harbor. The young man landed awkwardly in the water and drowned. When news spread of Griffin's tragic death, donors added another $50,000 in donations to fight ALS.

The Frates family was devastated. Pete took to Facebook and eulogized his longtime friend. "Team Frate Train lost a good friend today, Corey Griffin," Pete wrote. "Helping out was nothing new for Griff. . . . He worked his butt off these last few weeks for ALS. We texted every day, planning, and scheming ways to raise funds and plan events. . . . God Bless. RIP Corey."

Pete would find himself fighting for survival just a few months later, when he became stricken with pneumonia and had to be intubated in the hospital. Doctors placed a tube down his throat, which was taped to his mouth. The procedure was excruciatingly painful for Pete.

"He was so heavily medicated due to the discomfort of the tube that he wasn't able to communicate with me," Julie recalls. "No one should ever see a loved one intubated."

The family had a meeting with Pete's intensive-care doctor a few days after the procedure. Julie was exhausted after having spent the past seventy-two hours by her husband's bedside. She was joined at the meeting by John and her father, Joe. The question on the table was whether Pete would be willing to undergo a permanent tracheostomy. The operation would allow him to continue breathing through a ventilator and so extend his life. Surgeons would need to cut into Pete's neck just below the Adam's apple and through his windpipe and the cartilage rings along the outer walls. Doctors would then create a hole wide enough to stick a tracheostomy tube inside. Once the tube was hooked up to a ventilator, the machine would breathe for Pete. It would be a game changer for his health care. Doctors informed the family that only 10 percent of all ALS patients choose to go on a ventilator because it is not an easy road and many aspects of the care are not covered by health insurance. There are serious physical risks as well. An infection to the area around Pete's throat or excessive bleeding could kill him quickly. Despite these potential hazards, surgery was still his only hope.

"Either we place the trache in Pete, or he won't survive much longer," the intensive-care doctor said.

Julie already knew what Pete's decision would be. She had had the conversation with him many times before. Her husband had told her that he was willing to do whatever it took and submit to the highest levels of pain to stay alive for her and their new baby.

But how can I make such a life-altering decision for someone, my husband, the love of my life, without being able to talk to him now, just before the procedure? Julie asked herself.

The nurses decreased Pete's medication just enough for him to open his eyes and listen to Julie as she explained what was about to happen. "It's time to get that new necklace we talked about. Everything is going to be all right," she said, staring into his eyes.

Julie was not sure whether Pete heard her or not, but he knew she was there. The nurses quickly sedated him again, and the doctors performed the operation.

"The scene was horrific, my husband with a tube down his throat and moaning out in pain," she recalls. It was too much to take. Julie collapsed on the floor of the hospital room and sobbed. Nurses had to escort her out of the room, while John and Joe remained by Pete's side.

While all of this was happening, Pete's mother was halfway around the world, about to make an appearance on a popular television program in Stockholm, Sweden. When she spoke to John during a layover in London, her husband told her that Pete was not feeling well. During a follow-up call, Nancy learned that Pete had been admitted to Mass General Hospital.

"It's nothing major," John told her at the time. "We'll be out of here soon."

A brutal winter nor'easter was making its way to New England, and John saw no need for his wife to fly home and get trapped by the storm.

But now Pete was intubated and suffering from a serious bout with pneumonia. His health was dire, worse than anything the family had dealt with before. Julie spoke with Andrew and Jenn and learned that Nancy had not been informed of her son's grave condition. John thought he was doing the right thing by shielding her from the news that Pete was very sick. Julie and Jenn decided they needed to call her. "She is Pete's mom, and Jenn and I agreed that as mothers we could not imagine being so far away from our child in such a seriously life-threatening scenario," Jenn explained.

The women took the burden off John's shoulders and called Nancy from the hospital. "Mom, we are calling not as your daughters; we are calling as mothers," Julie and Jenn said over the phone. "Pete is really struggling, and we think you should come home."

Nancy took the next available flight back to Boston. When she arrived, Pete was in surgery.

"He's being put on a ventilator," the family told her.

Hours later, after he had woken up from surgery, Pete looked up at his family surrounding his bedside and he winked.

"It was his way of letting us know that it was going to be okay."

He spent four weeks in the hospital and in rehabilitation before returning home to Beverly with a full respiratory unit and a full-time respiratory nurse.

Pete was now on a feeding tube without the ability to swallow his own saliva or eat. He could no longer hold up his head, as the nerve cells in his brain and spine continued to die. Pete had finally lost all ability to speak.

"When the disease forced my son into silence, for me that was the toughest day since the diagnosis," Nancy recalls sadly. "I knew that I would never hear my darling son's voice again."

She now had to rely on her own fading memory: the high-pitched wail of a baby being born, his first words, the excitement in Pete's voice when he described playing his favorite sports, the night he urged his family not to mourn his diagnosis but to rally around him to find a cure.

"He would never say 'Mum' again," she says. "I would give anything for just one more conversation with my son."

Pete's once booming voice was now silent, and the only way that he could communicate was through a series of clicks and texts using his eye-gaze technology. The four main words used by Pete on a daily basis were *pee, poop, fan,* and *hands*. Yet through all the discomfort and pain, Pete continued to focus on the two things that made him happiest—his baby and baseball.

Daughter Lucy was growing into a healthy, happy child. "From the day we brought Lucy home from the hospital, the morning has always been Pete and Lucy time," Julie says. "Every morning I bring her into bed with us. When she was an infant I would lay her on his chest and wrap his arms around her. Now she snuggles right in under his arm. It has become both of their favorite parts of the day, as well as Lucy's 'safe place.' Whenever she is upset, tired, or scared, she asks to go in bed with Daddy. She knows that in that place, cuddled up next to her dad, that everything is okay."

Lucy began to roll, then crawl, and take those first steps with the balance and agility of her famous dad. Since Lucy was still very young and both were nonverbal, father and daughter shared a special bond, communicating through smiles and facial expressions. As soon as Lucy could walk, she began using her father's wheelchair as a jungle gym, climbing up the wheels and onto his lap to be closer to her daddy. His muscles could not respond to her touch, but his heart melted.

"I always joke with my friends that I may have a husband with ALS, but he spends more time with Lucy than most fathers spend with their kids," Julie says with a smile. "Her first words were *Da-da*. Her first steps were in our living room, being cheered on by Pete on his computer. He was there when she first tried solid food, and Pete laughed with me at the hilarious facial expressions of her first taste of sweet potato."

The only phrase Pete saved on his automated speaking program is "Lucy, Daddy loves you. Give me a kiss."

And there was still baseball. Ever since he was named director of Baseball Operations for Boston College following his 2012 diagnosis, Pete had served as the team's inspirational and motivational leader, whether he was physically with the team or not. Those first two seasons, Pete traveled to nearly every road game, but by 2015 he was physically unable to travel. But his connection to the program continued. The roster changed as players graduated and new players took the field, but the team's character remained the same. Upperclassmen watched Pete's struggles and triumphs with amazement, while the new kids learned about his story and their own roles in his expanding legacy. The players got to know Pete one on one, and when they needed a boost, they knew exactly who to turn to.

During the Eagles' stellar 2016 season, star shortstop Johnny Adams, of Walpole, Massachusetts, found himself struggling at the plate, so he asked Pete for advice through Facebook's messenger application. Pete offered tips on Adams's swinging technique, and the slugger soon got back on track.

While he was hitting under .200 at the season's halfway point, Adams snapped out of his slump and was one of the team's most lethal weapons, batting .370 for the rest of the season. The Eagles then went on a historic run, winning thirty-five games, the second-highest win total in school history. They were the Cinderella team entering the College World Series Tournament. The Eagles, as they had done since 2012, carried the Team Frate Train banner to every game, and Pete's presence was constant throughout the storybook season. As the underdog squad knocked off University of Utah and Tulane to advance to the final eight, the jubilant players called Pete via FaceTime from Coach Gambino's phone from the field, the locker room, or the team bus. Pete could not talk back, but he had a glint in his eye when the excited guys would come on the screen, saying, "Hey Pete, we love you man! We're doing this for you. Stay strong my brother!"

Boston College made it all the way to the College World Series Super Regional round, where they lost a three-game series to the third-ranked Miami Hurricanes. The Eagles were one game away from the college baseball semifinals and ended ranked sixteenth nationally, the highest in the program's history.

Pete loved watching that team, and, in many ways, their Cinderella season was a fitting capstone to Pete's dedication to changing the program from an afterthought to national recognition. While Pete's communication was mostly relegated to one-sentence tweets by that time, he was so proud of his Eagles that he mustered up the energy to do an interview with *Boston Herald* columnist Steve Buckley to sing their praises.

"Coming in to this year, I knew we would have a chance in the ACC tourney, but these boys totally bought in and are playing great with a ton of confidence … ahead of schedule but I'm not surprised at all," Pete messaged to Buckley. When asked why, Pete responded, "The culture cultivated by Mike and the staff has prepared these boys for this level of play. We don't whine, complain, or worry about external factors."

For Coach Gambino, Pete's influence extended far beyond the ball field. Through his actions and his words, Pete embodied the Jesuit spirit of Boston College and its motto: "Men and women for others."

"He's taught these boys who we want to be," Gambino said. "Yeah, it's about winning baseball games and becoming better players, but these are life lessons. When you have this guy who gets this diagnosis and his reaction is 'How can I help everyone else?' what better way to learn what it means to be a man or a woman for others? Pete is who all these boys want to be. He's a great father, a great husband, a man of character, and a man of integrity. He's the role model."

On May 7, 2016, Boston College saluted its former captain with the rarest of honors by retiring Pete's jersey number 3. His family and friends joined hundreds of supporters on a cold, damp day at Shea Field on the school's Chestnut Hill campus for the team's fifth annual ALS Awareness game against Wake Forest. Little Lucy, now a precocious bright-eyed toddler, was draped head to toe in maroon and gold, as was her father, who wore a Boston College baseball cap and blazer, with sneakers. Pete was lifted out of his customized van and wheeled onto the field by his brother, Andrew, and a caregiver, as players lined up outside their respective dugouts and cheered. In the distance, along the outfield wall hung two banners. The first banner number 13 honored Eddie Pellegrini, the winningest baseball coach in Boston College history. The banner stood alone for nearly twenty years until this day, when Pete would become only the second member of the BC baseball team to have his number retired. As the banner, emblazoned with a bright, bold number 3 was unveiled, the crowd broke out in thunderous applause. For many, their clapping was accompanied by tears. The man most overwhelmed by the gesture was Pete's father, John.

"Long before he became a worldwide symbol of a horrific disease, Pete was a baseball player," John said, during a quiet moment after the ceremony. "That's all he ever wanted to be known for in this life, and thanks to Boston College, he'll be remembered here on this field for the next hundred years as just that: a baseball player."

Athletes-turned–ALS warriors like Pete Frates and Steve Gleason had become global symbols for the cause. They had taken the torch lit by Lou Gehrig, Steve Heywood, and others, whose public battles with the insidious disease created a better understanding of ALS and the dire need to find a cure. Now it was time to hand the torch to others, younger and healthier than themselves, to turn hope into reality once and for all. The Frates family had recently met one such prospect. His name was Scott Matzka, a newly diagnosed University of Michigan hockey player who reminded John Frates a lot of his son.

Scott was a thirty-eight-year-old, married father of two beautiful children from Port Huron, Michigan, who had been diagnosed with ALS in 2015. He had won a national championship with the University of Michigan Wolverines in 1998, ironically over the Frates' beloved Boston College Eagles. In fact, it was Scott who assisted on the game-winning goal in overtime against the Eagles at Boston Garden, then called the Fleet Center, to win the title.

Scott had kept his diagnosis private between him and his wife, Catie, and called John before going public. In doing his research on how to fight the disease and raise awareness, Scott was amazed by Pete and reached out to John for some advice.

"He told me all about his illness, his symptoms," John recalled. "Every time I talk to a newly diagnosed patient, I know the path they are going to go down. I ask them to please join us. Nancy and I can go across the country and talk, but we're not the patient. The patient has the most effective voice, but it's limited."

Scott told John the same stories of how Pete discovered his illness. He was having trouble buttoning his shirt. His hands cramped and went numb. It was like déjà vu. In Scott, John saw a potential successor to Pete, who had many of the same qualities: a beautiful, loving family; a massive support network; an athletic background with an army of locker room buddies ready to help; and bold leadership skills. It was the same narrative as Pete, except instead of baseball, Scott's story was hockey.

John and Scott talked about social media and how to use his athletic connections to raise awareness. They talked about how the hockey-crazed area of Detroit and the U-Michigan hockey boosters and alumni could help, just as Boston and the Boston College family had embraced Pete.

"Scott, you have to formulate a plan and get out there," John told him. "You've unfortunately been given a terminal illness. You've unfortunately only got two to five years of strength. We're on the same team. Unfortunately, we've been selected for this team. Pete's been silenced. It's your time to carry the torch. Now it's your turn."

Those words stuck with Matzka, and when it came time to name his foundation, he called it My Turn. The foundation focuses on raising money for ALS patients, who incur an estimated $250,000 per-year care bill. "It's my turn to broadcast awareness and create a group behind me that will do the same," Matzka told the Michigan hockey website GoBlue. com. "One day, when I'm gone, that there will hopefully be a foundation that carries on the mission.

"John Frates told me to raise money for the cost of the disease and the effect it can have on a family. Eventually, I'll lose my ability to breathe on my own and will need a ventilator if I want to live, and a speaking tube. That home health care isn't covered by insurance, and so John said, 'We have to raise money. And when we do that, raise more.' So, our focus is to raise money for the families." Matzka has done just that, through several fund-raisers in Michigan and Illinois.

18

THE GREAT FLOOD

He wanted a swimming pool. That is why Dr. Michael Collins got into medicine. Collins, the esteemed chancellor of University of Massachusetts Medical School, was raised in the blue-collar town of Walpole, Massachusetts, where the only person who owned a swimming pool was the local doctor. Collins passed the doctor's home each day on his way to an after-school job at a paper store. *Someday, I'm gonna buy that house*, he told himself.

He scored good-enough grades to earn a place at a local private school, before going off to college at Holy Cross in Worcester, Massachusetts. His plan was to continue on to medical school and return to Walpole as the town doctor. Those plans were interrupted when his father was diagnosed with a brain tumor while the son was a sophomore in college. Michael Collins watched his father die an agonizing death, and that is when his career path took a different route. Now he wanted to help cure diseases instead of taking care of the everyday ailments of an entire community.

Collins received his medical training at Tufts Medical School and then went on to Texas Tech University, where he soon became the youngest medical school dean in the United States. He eventually came back to Massachusetts to head up the second-largest health-care system in New England before getting recruited by the University of Massachusetts Medical School. Collins then set about on a mission to change the course of history of disease. But for this, he would have to rely on grant funding from the National Institutes of Health (NIH).

The year was 2008, and while the U.S. military was apparently drawing down troops in the war in Iraq after a surge, there was no slowdown on the horizon to the bloody conflict in Afghanistan. Collins paid close attention to this, primarily because high military costs came at the expense of other governmental projects, including funding to fight disease.

"We spent $4 trillion on the war in Afghanistan," Collins says with disgust. "People like me had bought the government line that there wasn't enough funding for medical research, which had not seen an increase since 2002."

While the money was not there, at least not for medical and scientific research, the minds were. One of the brightest minds in the country belonged to Dr. Robert "Bob" Brown of Harvard University. Brown had actually mentored Pete Frates's ALS doctor Merit Cudkowicz, and, like her, he had dedicated his professional life to finding a cure for ALS. In 1993 he led a team of researchers that discovered the first gene linked to the inherited form of the disease. They named the gene SOD1. Bob Brown was considered a triple threat. He had the ability to perform science, he had a comforting bedside manner when caring for patients, and he could teach and lead.

Michael Collins's first mission as chancellor was to lure Brown away from Harvard to UMass Medical School. Dr. Brown toured the medical school campus and was excited to see such a collaborative environment. Researchers and students alike were starstruck by his presence. But Dr. Brown had a unique way of relaxing and reassuring folks to make them feel less intimidated by his brilliance. He was a folksy, plain talker, just like Chancellor Collins was.

"I don't want to waste your time or mine," Collins told him. "We have a vision here, which is to change the course of history of disease, and it seems that you're onto something with ALS."

Brown nodded in agreement. "Chancellor Collins, I'm fifty-eight years old, and every waking moment of my life, I want to cure ALS," he replied. "I don't know whether it's going to be stem-cell biology or gene therapy. But I do know that the finest place I can go is right here."

Bob Brown joined UMass Medical School and quickly went to work on the SOD1 gene. Before long he and his team discovered that the gene, which was connected to 20 percent of inherited or familial cases of the disease, had also shown up in cases of sporadic ALS. This was considered a breakthrough. If Brown's team could find a therapy to treat the rarest cases of this rare disease, that therapy could then be applied to the majority of people suffering from ALS.

—

In early January 2011 Chancellor Collins was greeted by a special visitor and longtime friend, former Massachusetts governor Paul Cellucci. In 1997, while serving as governor, Cellucci had signed a bill to create a $40 million medical research complex that would eventually become home to Dr. Brown's research lab. The lifelong Republican had been out of public life for a few years since resigning as U.S. ambassador to Canada under President George W. Bush in 2005. He had always been considered handsome. Many compared Cellucci's looks to that of Oscar-winning actor Robert De Niro. But on this day, he appeared haggard, thin, and sick. "I have ALS," he told Collins. "This is a terrible thing, but we want to do some good with it. I don't know if it'll help me, but we want to raise money for a cure. Are you with me, Michael?"

It was an offer the chancellor could not refuse. Governor Cellucci and his wife, Jan, secured Collins's partnership in creating the UMass ALS Cellucci Fund with a goal to raise $10 million for research under the direction of Dr. Bob Brown. The money would allow Brown and his colleagues to seize the moment and chase after medical breakthroughs immediately rather than being forced to wait years for traditional funding.

"We then met with a few marketing agencies to figure out how we could tap into social media for crowd funding," Collins recalls. "We just weren't inspired enough to come up with a solution."

Donations to the Cellucci fund reached about half its goal, as the former governor's health got progressively worse. In late May 2013 Cellucci called the chancellor at his office. His once-commanding voice was now as soft as a whisper. "I don't want you to give up," Cellucci told Collins. "I want you to keep going. I may not be able to do this much longer, but

I want you to give me your word that you're gonna continue at this and that we're gonna work hard to find a cure for ALS. You need to see this through."

Paul Cellucci died one month later. The chancellor was devastated. The two men had become particularly close. When Cellucci was asked to throw out the first pitch before a Red Sox game at Fenway Park in the spring of 2011, he asked Collins to perform the honor for him, as he was now too weak to grip and throw a baseball. Democrat Deval Patrick, the governor at the time, had declared the day as Paul Cellucci/ALS Champion Day in the commonwealth of Massachusetts. Now, two years later, Cellucci was dead and not much had changed.

"He took on this fight with such dignity and grace and never once thought of himself," Collins says. "He deserved better." Once again, the chancellor compared the numbers. "Do the math on $4 trillion. Ten percent of $4 trillion is $300 billion. $300 billion is what the NIH allocates for research funding over a ten-year period. That's only 10 percent of what we spent on the war in Afghanistan."

ALS patients like Governor Cellucci and Pete Frates were fighting a different war at home, a war against an invisible enemy that had staked a claim on their bodies and refused to negotiate. For the insidious disease, victory could only come in death.

"We are losing a whole generation of America's best scientists," says Collins. "Our research armies have been depleted because the best and brightest are forced into other fields due to lack of funding."

In August of the following year, Collins was driving with his assistant when he heard something crazy on the radio. A local television reporter had challenged him to dump a bucket of ice water on his head. "That's the dumbest thing I've ever heard," Collins shouted.

His assistant reached into his pocket and fished for his iPhone. "Chancellor, that may not be so dumb," the assistant told him. They pulled to the side of the road, and the assistant played a video clip on his phone. "Here's your son doing the Ice Bucket Challenge. And here's your daughter doing the same thing."

It was so brilliant in its simplicity. Yet the idea had escaped a room full of social-media gurus Collins consulted with in the past.

"Are you gonna do it?" the assistant asked.

"It's not exactly my style," the chancellor replied. "But if I'm willing to do this, how many others will join?"

Dr. Michael Collins, esteemed leader of the most prestigious medical research school in the United States, accepted the Ice Bucket Challenge. The next day he stood in the center of campus with Dr. Bob Brown. "We got your challenge," Collins said on video. "We have the challenge every day of looking after people with ALS. We appreciate the fact that you've called us out. We challenge your viewers to make a donation to the UMass Cellucci ALS Fund."

Chancellor Collins says that what the Ice Bucket Challenge did for him was to show that people want research. "The American spirit can be defined as a freedom to choose your own destiny," he says. "We can do whatever we set out to do. The people said, 'We want research, and not only do we want it, we will pay for it.' The Ice Bucket Challenge was equivalent to a great flood that threatens the town. Everyone grabs sandbags and runs to help."

Professor John Landers always wanted to help people. While in tenth grade in Albany, New York, he took his first biology class and he loved it. From that time forward, he knew exactly what he wanted to do with his life. His father was a social studies teacher, and his mother was a banquet server. There were no scientists in his family. He graduated at the top of his class in high school and then sailed through college at Rensselaer Polytechnic Institute and entered the University of Pennsylvania, where he studied molecular biology and performed cancer research as he worked toward his doctorate. His research career eventually led him to MIT in Cambridge, Massachusetts, where he worked to develop new ways to analyze DNA. These were the days before the groundbreaking discovery of the human genome, which contains all the genetic information in a person. There are roughly three billion genetic differences between the average two people. Landers and his team were tasked with analyzing those differences, but there was no easy way to do it, so his team created a process where they could analyze many different variants all at the same time. The plan was successful.

In 1998 Landers formed his own small biotech company in Worcester and continued the work there. He ran out of money when the biotech bubble burst and the attacks of September 11, 2001, turned off the spigots for serious research funding. He returned to the world of genetic academics. That is when he met Dr. Robert Brown and was lured into the challenging world of ALS research. Eventually, Landers the researcher joined Brown the clinician at UMass Medical.

"At the time I didn't know a whole lot about ALS genetics," Landers says. "No one knew a lot about it. What I did know was that ALS is a horrific disease that destroys entire families, so I learned as much as I could."

Admittedly, Landers did not know much about social media. He had spent his free time touring amusement parks and riding roller coasters with his son. He had no idea what the Ice Bucket Challenge was or when it began. Soon, colleagues and friends were filling him in about the Internet sensation.

"As more and more people did it, I said, 'Wow, this is real,'" Landers recalls. "I ended up doing it as well, right out in front of our building. It took off like wildfire. I had never seen anything else like it." Still, it would take some time for the online conflagration to have a direct impact on Landers's world. His life's work was one that required great patience. "Oftentimes, you never see the benefit of what you are working on," he says.

So Landers and his ten-person team, which included three members of a family of scientists from Dublin, Ireland, continued their work slowly and methodically, because what they were looking for could not be easily found.

"Imagine that someone walked into a room with 5,500 copies of Leo Tolstoy's epic tome *War and Peace* and dumped them on the floor," Landers explains. "And they told you that there was one misspelled word on one page of one copy of the 1,225 page book and that your job is to find it. That's what we do. We have to find that one change that is occurring in that patient. We have to find that new gene."

They were looking for that needle in a haystack. To seize the moment and spark a breakthrough, Landers needed pennies from heaven. What he got instead was something even more significant. His team received a $1 million grant from the ALS Association. The research windfall was made possible by Pete Frates and the Ice Bucket Challenge. Landers used the grant to team up with Dr. Jan Veldink, his counterpart at the University Medical Center Utrecht in the Netherlands. Together they began work to identify all the genes that cause both hereditary (familial) and sporadic ALS.

The team discovered a gene it later named NEK1. The gene had several different functions in neurons. The particular genetic variation was present in 3 percent of all cases of both hereditary and sporadic ALS in Europe as well as North America. It was as close to a eureka moment as one could imagine in the painstaking field of ALS research. By identifying the new NEK1 gene, which may contribute to the cause of ALS, Landers and his team now hope they will be able to develop a therapy to treat the deadly disease. News of the scientific discovery and its connection to the Ice Bucket Challenge made headlines around the world.

Drug makers were also making strides. Nancy Frates spoke at a pharmaceutical research conference in Washington, DC, in 2015 and implored the nation's top executives and researchers to give ALS patients and their families the chance they deserve: "When you go back to your companies, put ALS on the table for discussion."

One researcher in the audience later wrote Nancy that she had taken a new job with a company that was as committed as she was to the fight against ALS. In August 2016 that company, Mitsubishi Tanabe Pharma Corporation, announced from its Osaka, Japan, headquarters that the U.S. Food and Drug Administration had accepted the company's application for a new intravenous drug, edaravone, which is believed to relieve the effects of oxidative stress brought on by unstable molecules, a likely factor in the progression of ALS.

After four long years of raising more than $220 million and traveling the globe to increase awareness, the Frates family felt the battle had finally begun to shift and that researchers were slowly gaining the upper hand against amyotrophic lateral sclerosis. Their efforts and the efforts of millions the world over could help save the lives of all ALS patients in the decades to come. It could become a treatable disease and even a curable one.

But Pete, the brave young man who had led the charge, was no longer fighting the global war against ALS. He was fighting for himself and for his family and was struggling to live every second of every day.

19

INSPIRATION

Pete was alive, but he was not living. As the summer of 2016 wore on, his health continued to deteriorate to the point where he was staying in bed all day and not interacting with the two most important people in his life—Julie and Lucy. He had developed sepsis and was gravely ill. The family rushed him to Mass General Hospital, where they kept vigil over him for several days. Pete was in excruciating pain and barely hanging on.

Like all those closest to Pete, his sister, Jenn, had watched helplessly for weeks as he grew weaker and more withdrawn. The latest infection had triggered a fever and made it even more difficult for Pete to breathe. It was at that point that Jenn felt she needed to have the one conversation with Pete that no one else could. She dropped off her children at John and Nancy's and drove to the hospital. A nurse was attending to Pete when she entered his room. Jenn asked the nurse to leave the room for a moment. She reached for a chair and dragged it next to his bed and sat down. She took his hand in hers.

"Pete, I know you're suffering, and I know you're sick. I know you're putting on a brave face for everybody," Jenn said tearfully. "But if you need to go, it is okay. It's okay to go now. I want you to know that we will take care of Julie and Lucy."

Pete stared at his sister intently. Jenn started sobbing heavily. He looked to his notepad and began typing with his eyes. "All my peeps, thx for da love," he wrote, sending the message via Twitter, for the world to see. "im doin fine. med weed and netflix. oh ya, for all the worrywarts out there, never forget how effn tuff i am."

Pete was angry and that was a good thing. Jenn had awoken her brother's fierce competitive spirit. At that moment, he began the long fight back. If he was going to be here on Earth, he was going to be present.

"He flipped the infection right on its head," Jenn recalls. "He was going to beat it. He was going to win."

Pete regained his strength and got better. Soon he was out of the hospital and back home. He did it through sheer will.

———

The fall proceeded at a frenetic pace for the Frates clan. There was of course the usual day-to-day schedule juggling with nurses and family members, all focused on carving out time to care for Pete, as well as the normal hustle and bustle of a busy family household.

While the focus had always been raising awareness of ALS and finding treatments and cures, caring for Pete by now had become priority number one as his condition worsened. With Pete's lack of mobility and declining health, caring for him had now become a full-time job, not only for the nurses and doctors who keep him alive, but also for Julie, John, Nancy, Andrew, and Jenn, in addition to countless other friends and relatives. It became a chaotic symphony of coming and going, with Nancy traveling around the country raising awareness for the deadly disease slowly consuming her son.

Nancy had emerged as a national figure in the ALS fight. In the fall of 2016 alone, she traveled to Chicago and San Francisco for motivational speeches. She also spoke at a women's forum at her alma mater, Boston College, and was appointed to the board of trustees at Endicott College in their hometown of Beverly. The school just a few weeks earlier had dedicated an entire new residence hall in Pete's name, adorned with murals and inspirational photos of Pete, Lou Gehrig, and the Ice Bucket Challenge.

While Nancy traveled and Julie took care of little Lucy, John and Andrew stepped up to handle a lot of the day-to-day duties with Pete, helping the nurses move him around and clean, shave and dress him. John and

Andrew give each other tips, seemingly almost daily, as Pete's needs shift. What works one day does not necessarily work the next.

Moving Pete from his bed to his wheelchair, showering him, helping him go to the bathroom, and getting him as comfortable as possible was a constant battle. When they first had to start shaving Pete, there were disagreements, as Andrew shaved only going up, while Pete liked to shave up and down. He also always used a hot towel and lotion before his shave.

"He's a stubborn dude," Andrew joked.

At first, it was uncomfortable, as John struggled with having to help his oldest son perform the most personal tasks—things parents should never have to do for their children once they are out of diapers. But soon it became routine, as it was the family's "new normal."

The season also provided some relief for Andrew, as he had seven friends' weddings to attend, including some in which he was a member of the bridal party. It was also a time of transition for him, as he got a new job at a celebrity-marketing company run by ex–Boston Bruin Cleon Daskalakis, and a new girlfriend, Alycia Dell'Orfano, a striking brunette who happened to go to high school in Marblehead with Julie. He was living in South Boston, not far from where his brother once lived in his post–Boston College days, and met Alycia on the popular online dating site Bumble.

There was an immediate attraction, but also a strong bond right from the start. Like Andrew, Alycia knew the pain of watching a sibling suffer. Her only sister, Brianna, died of brain cancer when she was nine years old and Alycia was just six. Alycia has a small tattoo of her sister's name on her wrist. Andrew and Alycia went on their first date in July 2016 at Trade, a Boston waterfront hotspot. The normal first-date awkwardness was there, but they quickly felt comfortable enough with each other to share the stories of their siblings.

"We understand each other in a way that a lot of people can't," Alycia said.

She quickly became part of the Frates' extended family, accompanying Andrew to the ALS gala and other fund-raisers and joining the rotating cast of loved ones at the Beverly home. Starting a new relationship and job is difficult enough, but Andrew was constantly feeling guilty about not being home more for Pete. It was John who sat down with his son and told him to take a bit of a break and that he would pick up the slack. "I'm an old man; I've already lived my life," John told his son. "You have got to get out and live. I'll take care of this."

The stresses manifested themselves daily, as normal family disagreements erupted into full-blown shouting matches. Each family member had to remind themselves of the bigger picture whenever the stress got to be too much.

"The disease is so awful," Andrew says. "We're in such a tough spot. We're all worried about each other. Everyone is trying to handle it the best we can. Your moods change so much."

As had been the case in the family for years, Pete was often the voice of reason or the one who knocked everyone back into line.

Nancy often sat by Pete's bedside, hugging him and kissing him, giving him medical advice or telling him to get out of bed. Some days Pete did not want all the fuss and kicked her out of the room. The same happened with John, as Pete's frustration spilled over at times, and he just wanted to be alone.

"It became like a sports locker room," says Andrew. "You say what you have to say, process it, and move on."

Medically, every day posed a new challenge, as Pete's condition grew direr by the hour. His care had moved to the palliative stage, which is similar to hospice and focused on making a terminal patient comfortable at home. With winter coming the family was warned that Pete was highly susceptible to pneumonia and other infections and could land back in the hospital at any moment. He had constant lung infections that were treated with antibiotics. His bladder, like the rest of his muscles and organs, had shut down, leaving him vulnerable to urinary tract infections. As a result, his bladder needed to be emptied by catheter every three hours. He would have spasms. He was close to the "locked-in phase," a term used to describe ALS patients who are literally a prisoner in their own body with no ability to move or communicate. Pete was close, they said ominously. Within months.

A family therapist came once a week, including a counselor who would try and talk to Pete about his end-of-life wishes. But Pete would not talk about it. He refused to think in those terms. It was an agonizing position, as Pete was convinced he would be cured.

"He thought the phone is going to ring in the next hour and someone would tell him, 'We've got the pill. We've got the injection,'" John somberly explained. "He thinks he's going to get up out of that chair and walk like the last five years never happened."

Another harsh blow to the family came in early November, when the family got their October medical bill: $88,000. The staggering figure was double what Pete's monthly care had been. It went from roughly $40,000 a month to $60,000 to now almost $90,000. Much of it is attributed to the escalating care needed to keep Pete alive and comfortable, and now that he was in palliative care at home little, if any, was covered by insurance.

Most of his medications were experimental or not FDA approved, so they were paid for out of pocket by the family. One drug alone—a saliva-producing medication that allows Pete to swallow—costs $6,000 a month and is not covered because it is considered experimental. An experimental cystic fibrosis treatment medication his doctors recommended cost another $5,000 a month. Up to this point, the family had spent roughly $1.5 million in roughly two-and-a-half years of escalating care.

The staggering spend rate prompted an emergency family meeting to discuss finances and strategy. Pete's foundation, the Pete Frates #3 Fund, covered much of Pete's care but asking donors to continue to contribute was becoming a burden. The family had a frank, very tense conversation about how to proceed. Things got heated.

"Pete should be a part of this," Nancy said.

"That's ridiculous," John says. "Don't do that."

Julie was the voice of reason and made a ruling: "He does not have to be involved." They all nodded in agreement. Julie was right. They all knew that Pete would be devastated if he knew they were fighting about money to care for him.

Still, the family had some realistic questions to answer: Can we raise any more money? How can we cut costs? One way was to bring in more caregivers rather than nurses. Nurses generally cost a hundred dollars an hour, while caregivers are about twenty-five dollars an hour. The problem was that much of Pete's care required nurses at that point. And because he was at home, and not hospitalized, all the cost of the nurses was out of the family's pocket. John and Nancy feared the tab would soon be over $100,000 a month.

They decided to send out a plea letter to Pete's biggest donors, letting them know of the dire circumstances and asking for help. They also decided to have a follow-up meeting with the nursing supervisor to discuss options. They asked if there were any ways to reduce rates. The nursing company is a for-profit enterprise, but they had been close to the family for years now, so they were very compassionate and amenable to working with the distraught clan.

It was decided the family could go on a payment plan and that care would continue, regardless of the family's ability to pay the monthly tab. "We won't abandon Pete," the supervisor assured John.

Pete knew the situation was dire and, despite his diminishing ability to communicate, he knew this was a pivotal moment for the family. So he dug deep and sent the following message to the family: (NOTE: This message is printed exactly as Pete sent it. By this point, Pete communicated solely through Twitter and Facebook Messenger, spelling out words with his eyes. His eye-movement ability had decreased significantly, which is why there are so many spelling and grammar errors.)

PETE: ok folk. i hvnt needed to giv a pep tlsinc mrch of -2012 for years u hv been crshing it!

we hv cnhngd our lil disees frevr! bt it is time to regroup gtj get the teem togthr for!

our bggst push yet! i propose 3-prongd attack! 1. our reg, events, ampd up ,foc

PETE: hyprgfovud on hyprfocusd on fundrai.com

PETE: two.,. . lrettr wrtng campaign ftom ,mr from me,juli,luvy to top tipytop donords!

ANDREW chimed in, saying, "Yes. I think that needs to be the focus. Dad and I can help with the wording."

PETE: "akathree. . huge, evnt in boston celebs,politicians,etc. lts meet to discuss asap . . . thx! n

go!"

He also gave a list of the top corporate and sports sponsors they should reach out to for this big fund-raising push. John says writing this message took all of Pete's strength over a day or two.

The next message came from Nancy: "You amaze me! You know we will get it done! I LOVE YOU PETE FRATES!"

Throughout all the madness, uncertainty, and challenges around him, Pete somehow maintained his leadership in the family and continued to exhibit all the qualities that made him such a magnetic personality. In the fall of 2016, he grew a man-bun and then a man-ponytail—initially to Julie's chagrin, but soon she grew to love it. He posted pictures on social media wearing Lou Gehrig socks and red-white-and-blue Sperry shoes. He continued to be a prolific tweeter, posting frequently during the Chicago Cubs historic World Series run, offering droll political commentary during President Trump's rise to power, and hailing his pal Red Sox slugger David Ortiz upon his retirement.

"Pete has a healthy ego; there's no doubt about it. ALS has taken everything from him except his ego," John says. "It was never cockiness. It was a good healthy belief in himself."

Pete's tweets, at this point, were the only real window into his mind and heart, as his communication had become extremely limited. In addition to using his retina screen, Pete managed to communicate with his family through his eyes. Andrew said he could tell what Pete wanted or was thinking with a simple look. If he and the caregivers were discussing moving Pete or how to position him, a look from Pete would always confirm what Pete wanted. Andrew was not sure exactly how it worked, if it was brotherly instinct or something deeper, but it was real.

But Pete's eyes were slowing down. The doctors in early November told the family that his eyes were down to just 20 percent usage and that the family should expect them to cease working soon. It was a monumental blow to the family, as they were all too aware that once Pete's eye movement stopped, so too would his ability to communicate in any way.

His diminishing abilities did not stop his thirst for adventure, however. In September Pete took it upon himself to have a TV and DVD player installed in the custom van that he travels in. No one knew about it until a nurse came up to John one day and said, "What are you doing tomorrow? Pete bought this system with video, a backup camera, [and] Bluetooth, and it needs to be installed. It's going to require a day or two at Best Buy."

It was classic Pete. Here everyone is worrying themselves sick about Pete's health and level of care, and he's buying toys.

One adventurous day Pete decided to try out the new system. Andrew was at his job at Celebrity Marketing, near the Boston Garden, when he got a random text from Pete.

"Dude, get some B's tix," Pete said.

The Bruins had been extremely generous to the Frates family, always accommodating Pete for games and pitching in with charitable endeavors, especially Hall of Famer Ray Bourque, Pete's boyhood idol who had become a close friend of the family. The Bruins arranged tickets for Ray's suite for Pete, Andrew, and some friends.

On the way there Pete had Andrew put a new AC/DC live concert video on the van's system. They rolled out of Beverly and down I-93 toward the Garden with "For Those about to Rock" blaring from the speakers and screen. Andrew may or may not have put a beer or two in Pete's feeding tube. Pete could not smile, but his eyes told Andrew he was happy.

The Bruins lost 5–0 that night to the Minnesota Wild but it was a memorable night, nonetheless, and a welcome break from the ALS stress for the brothers.

In December 2016 the NCAA presented Pete Frates with another major honor, its 2017 Inspiration Award. Normally, the recipient accepts the award at the NCAA's annual January gala in Nashville, Tennessee, but because of Pete's progressing disease, Mark Emmert, the organization's president, made a house call to the Frates home in Beverly. The spacious home was made smaller, as throngs of well-wishers, including Pete's grandparents, friends, and former coaches, crowded into the living room for the official presentation. Moments later a bus packed with Boston College baseball players rolled into the neighborhood and parked outside. The players and Coach Gambino walked single file into the house and stood at attention waiting for their inspirational leader.

There was a moment of panic for Julie when she could not find Lucy in her bedroom or in the living room among the dozens of well-wishers.

Julie rushed into her own bedroom to find Lucy perfectly positioned with her favorite blanket, in bed cuddled up next to Pete. The scene next door was chaotic with television cameras and strange people, so the child retreated to her safe place, close to her father.

Lucy watched as John and Andrew got Pete dressed. Once again Pete called for his maroon-and-gold blazer. As reporters and photographers took their place, Pete was wheeled into the crowded room. The family's kitchen table had to be moved to accommodate the event. It was the same table in the same room where Pete Frates had, on the worst day of his life, made a pledge to change the world. On this day he would be honored for inspiring college athletes at Boston College and across the United States. But everyone present understood that his achievements were much greater.

Pete had organized the world's biggest bucket brigade. He brought people closer together despite differences of race, religion, creed, or color. At a time in human history where it appeared that the world had gone mad and divisiveness was the only commonality, he reminded people of the pure goodness in their hearts and the goodness in others. The Ice Bucket Challenge was not just a social-media campaign; it was a campaign of the human spirit. And as his body grew weaker, his spirit grew stronger. NCAA president Emmert summed up the feelings of everyone who had ever met Pete Frates and the millions around the world who have come to know him through witnessing the greatest and most difficult challenge of his life: "For all you've done and continue to do for humanity, thank you so much."

The award was placed on Pete's lap, the dead muscles in his arms and hands refusing to allow him to touch it. While holding Lucy in one arm, Julie smiled at her husband and ran her warm hand across his forehead. "Pete said from the moment he was diagnosed that he was going to change the trajectory of this disease, and that's exactly what he's done," his wife said.

John added, "One man can change the world. He inspired a movement that is the largest viral sensation in the history of mankind so that we never have to hear those three letters ALS again."

In his 2014 article for MLB.com, honoring the seventy-fifth anniversary of Lou Gehrig's farewell address, Pete saw promise for the future: "I want the *100th* anniversary of Lou Gehrig's speech to be a celebration of a courageous man who became the poster boy for a disease with a cure, not a cruel reminder of how nothing has changed in a century."

After the NCAA-award ceremony, one of his old baseball coaches in attendance offered these words: "It's known as Lou Gehrig's disease, but it will be known as Pete Frates's cure."

———

Pete is drawn to the sea. It provides him with strength and blessings. He had met the love of his life on the ocean; he had celebrated the news of impending fatherhood here. And on this day, New Year's 2017, he returned to the sea once again with his family and nearly two hundred friends, supporters, and strangers who were as committed as he was to life. All had gathered for the fifth annual Plunge for Pete swim at Good Harbor Beach in Gloucester, Massachusetts. The sun shined brightly, and the temperatures hinted at a coming thaw. Pete sat in his wheelchair near ocean's edge, wrapped in a blanket and comforted by the warmth of those around him. As participants faced winter's rush of cold water, something else caught Pete's eye. It was his beautiful and fearless wife, Julie, taking a mother-daughter stroll with Lucy. He was not supposed to be here to witness this. The life expectancy of an ALS patient is two to five years. In March 2017 Pete would reach that five-year ceiling. He should be in the final stages of a courageous life. His eyes were supposed to have ceased working already, ending his ability to communicate with the outside world. The scientific experts told the family so. But what cannot be described or quantified by any medical expert on any medical chart is the true measure of a human being. No doctor or scientist can x-ray what is in a person's heart or what is in a person's dreams.

Pete Frates has a dream. He imagines the day when he can free himself from his wheelchair and tubes, take fresh air into his lungs, stand up on a pair of strong legs, and walk Julie and Lucy to the ocean or back to the fields of dreams of his youth and show them where he developed the determination to overcome and the strength to be a champion of life. It is a dream that will never die, as his courageous spirit has inspired millions and proved that, yes, indeed, one man can change the world.

ACKNOWLEDGMENTS

CASEY SHERMAN   In January 2016 Boston-based sports-marketing executives Cleon Daskalakis and Christa Jones sat down to discuss their client and friend Nancy Frates and her family's dream of having a book written to chronicle their journey. Christa suggested me for this important literary endeavor, and I received a call soon after. At first, I resisted the challenge. My life was a whirlwind at the time, as Walt Disney Pictures was bringing my best-selling book *The Finest Hours* to the big screen, and I was crisscrossing the country, attending movie screenings and red-carpet premieres. I told them that I simply did not have the time needed to devote to the project. Daskalakis and Jones persisted and asked me to meet the Frates family at their Beverly home.

"At worst, you'll meet some wonderful people," Daskalakis said. "At best, you'll discover your next book project."

The only problem with that, I told him, was that I had just signed a deal for my next book project and would soon enter the research phase before writing. How could I pull this off? The answer was just a phone call away. Journalist Dave Wedge, my writing partner for our 2015 book, *Boston Strong: A City's Triumph over Tragedy*, had been eager to work on another project. Dave had read about the Frates family, as had I, and although we admired them greatly, we did not know whether their story could sustain a full narrative needed for a book like this. On a Sunday morning in February 2016, we drove together from our homes just south of Boston to the town of Beverly. We were interested in meeting them but remained noncommittal about moving ahead. As a writer of eight books, I usually know within five minutes of meeting someone whether or not there is enough compelling material for a book. When we were invited into the Frateses' home and met Nancy, John, Julie, Lucy, Andrew, and, most important, Pete, I knew in my heart within two minutes that we had to write this book. After you read *Challenge*, I know you will feel the same. Their story is about love—the love of a family committed to one another and committed to changing the world for good. Our initial meetings evolved into long interviews. Pete listened to each question and responded through his eye movement–reading scan. He was always honest in his responses and corrected his family when their recollections had faded with time. Pete was the sharpest person in the room, always.

The family allowed us into their tight-knit world, and we were given a window into their toughest moments and greatest triumphs. For this, we cannot thank the Frates family enough. They will continue to inspire us each and every day. We also give thanks to "the circles of Pete," that vast network of close friends and supporters who provided us with story after story of how Pete has changed their lives for the better. I would like to thank Cleon Daskalakis and Christa Jones for thinking of me. I would also like to thank Jennifer Berryman of the University of Massachusetts Medical School for connecting me with Chancellor Michael F. Collins, MD, and John Landers, PhD. These dedicated healers are the reason that ALS will one day be eradicated from this earth. Thanks go to Brian Frederick of the ALS Association for his time and insight. I would like to thank Dave Wedge, my writing partner and brother, for taking another emotional journey with me. We both shed tears of sadness for Pete's struggles and tears of joy for his personal victories. Thanks go to our Whydah Productions partner, Ted Collins; and to our film partner, Alison Greenspan of DiNovi Pictures. Thanks also go to our Hollywood reps, Ellen Goldsmith-Vein, Tony Gill, and Shari Smiley of Gotham Group, for believing in this project. I also thank my own family—daughters Isabella and Mia; their wonderful mom, Laura; my mother, Diane Dodd; my brother, Todd F. Sherman; and my uncle, Jim Sherman. Thank you all for your tremendous love and support. Most of all, I would like to thank

Pete Frates for showing us and the world what strength and courage truly look like.

January 2017

DAVE WEDGE   I would like to thank the entire Frates family for entrusting us to share Pete's story with the world. You inspired us every step of the way, and we continue to be amazed by your grace, passion, and love. I'd also like to thank the following people, in no particular order, for their assistance, cooperation, kindness, compassion, and inspiration in helping us tell this story: Tommy Haugh, Coach Pete Hughes, Coach Mike Gambino, Ryne Reynoso, Henry Pynchon, Carly Nardella, Pat Harrington, Ryan Tracy, Dylan Cox, Mike Pitt, Jack Dunn, Ed Hayward and the entire Boston College community, Scott Matzka, Pat Quinn and family, Steve Gleason, Meghan Hornblower, and Cleon Daskalakis. It has been a great privilege to tell this story, and it would not have been possible without the incredible support from my amazing wife, Jessica; Danielle and Jackson, the loves of my life; my dad, Roger; sisters Allyson and Nancy and the entire extended Wedge, Cornelius, and Heslam families; and all my friends and family from Brockton and Boston College. I'd also like to thank my editors and all my current and former colleagues at VICE; my reps at the Gotham Group and ZSH Literary; Alison Greenspan at DiNovi Pictures for her passion for this project; and all the researchers, families, and ALS warriors out there fighting this disease.

January 2017

THE FRATES FAMILY   We would like to thank Team Frate Train and the thousands of people who follow, support, and donate over and over again to Pete and our family. We would also like to thank our nuclear family and core group of friends, who unconditionally love and help us to provide as near normal a life as possible for us. We also thank our nurses and caregivers. They are a true gift from above who faithfully and lovingly devote their expertise and energies to Pete. We give our heartfelt thanks to ALS doctors, researchers, and clinicians. This amazing group is dedicated to solving the worst terminal disease, working tirelessly against insurmountable odds. It takes a very special person to go to work every day, knowing the batting average is .000 against ALS. We thank the city of Beverly, Massachusetts. You are the epicenter of love and support and exemplify an action city of helpers and doers. We also thank our St. John's Prep family. The spirituality and grace you have instilled in us have helped us shine a light on this disease to the world. We thank Boston College baseball and Head Coach Mike Gambino. From day one of the diagnosis to appointing Pete as director of baseball operations, you have done so much for our family. We thank Boston's professional sports teams for contributing tickets and game experiences to our events and accommodating Pete and his posse, whatever his needs are. We thank the MLB, commissioners Bud Selig and Rob Manfred, and executives Pat Courtney and Mike Teevan for embracing our cause and showing us that you "own" Lou Gehrig's disease. We thank the NCAA and President Mark Emmert for honoring Pete with the highest award a college athlete can achieve. We thank the Boston Red Sox for fulfilling the dream of this product of Massachusetts by signing Pete to a lifetime contract before a packed Opening Day crowd. We thank Steve Gleason, who demonstrates so beautifully how to live with ALS, for immediately accepting and mentoring Pete. And, finally, we thank Pat Quinn for passing along the simple act of dumping ice water over one's head for a cause and tagging Pete with one of his challenges, setting in motion the largest viral sensation in history—the ALS Ice Bucket Challenge.

January 2017

SOURCES

Brodeur, Nicole. "Former NFL player Steve Gleason on the Ice Bucket Challenge." *Seattle Times*, August 21, 2014.

Buckley, Steve. "Buckley: Ex-Eagle Pete Frates Won't Let ALS Dim His Passion for BC Baseball." *Boston Herald*, June 9, 2016.

Duplessy, Derrick. "Managing the Ice Bucket Challenge and Career Challenges with Lynn Aaronson." 2015. Podcast audio, 43.59. PurposeRockstar.com.

ESPN Sports Center. "Pete Frates: A Father's Legacy." Watertown, MA: DGA Productions, 2015. Video, 6:59. ESPN.com.

———. "Pete's Challenge." Watertown, MA: DGA Productions, 2014. Video, 7:00. YouTube.com.

Frates, Pete. "My Journey from Baseball Star to ALS Patient, 75 Years after Lou Gehrig." *Bleacher Report*, July 2, 2014.

Gallico, Paul. *Lou Gehrig: Pride of the Yankees*. New York: Open Road Media, 2015.

Kornacki, Steve. "Kornacki: Matzka Bringing Fight against ALS to Yost Ice Arena." October 6, 2016. MGoBlue.com.

Lou Gehrig's official website. Accessed March 30, 2017. LouGehrig.com.

Quinn, Pat. "Pat Quinn Talks ALS." Video, 1:23. August 20, 2014. MLB .com.

THE AUTHORS ASK THAT YOU PLEASE DONATE TO AN ALS CHARITY OF YOUR CHOICE.

Frates family (PeteFrates.com)

ALS Association (ALSA.org)

The Angel Fund (TheAngelFund.org)

ALS Therapy Development Institute (ALS.net)

UMass ALS Cellucci Fund (UMassMed.edu/Advancement/Ways-to-Give /Fundraising-Priorities/UMass-ALS-Cellucci-Fund/)

ABOUT THE AUTHORS

CASEY SHERMAN is an award-winning journalist and the *New York Times* best-selling author of *The Finest Hours* (now a major motion picture); *Boston Strong: A City's Triumph over Tragedy*, coauthored by Dave Wedge (an inspiration for the major motion picture *Patriots Day*); *Animal*; *A Rose for Mary*; *Bad Blood*; *Black Irish*; and *Black Dragon*. He is also a contributing writer for *Esquire* and *Boston* magazine and an international correspondent for FOX News. He is the cofounder of Whydah Productions and lives in Massachusetts. Follow him on Twitter @CaseySherman123 and on Facebook at Facebook.com/casey.sherman.

Sherman has appeared on hundreds of national and international television and radio programs and is a sought-after national speaker. He is represented by the APB Speakers Bureau and Gotham Group, Beverly Hills, California.

DAVE WEDGE is a best-selling author and writer based in Boston. A Boston College graduate, he writes for *VICE* and was an award-winning investigative reporter at the *Boston Herald* for fourteen years. He has also written for *Esquire*, *Newsweek*, and *DigBoston*, among other outlets. His first book, *Boston Strong: A City's Triumph over Tragedy*, about the 2013 Boston Marathon attacks and written with *New York Times* best-selling author Casey Sherman, was an inspiration for the 2016 film *Patriots Day*, starring Mark Wahlberg and directed by Peter Berg. He is also a partner in Whydah Productions and lives in Milton, Massachusetts, with his wife, *Boston Herald* columnist Jessica Heslam, and their children, Danielle and Jackson. Dave is represented by Gotham Group, Beverly Hills, California, and zsh Literary in New York City. Follow him on Twitter @DaveWedge.